The Only Two Causes of All Diseases: Achieve Longevity by Controlling the Hypothermia and Hypoxia!

Toru ABO

Professor, Medical Doctor
Department of Immunology School of Medicine
Niigata University

The Only Two Causes of All Diseases:
Achieve Longevity by Controlling the Hypothermia and
Hypoxia!

Published by Babel Press U.S.A.

This book was originally published in Japanese under the title
"人が病気になるたった2つの原因"
by Kodansha Ltd., Tokyo, Japan in 2010.

Author: Toru Abo

Supervisor: Mayumi Watanabe
Translator: Kyoko Shakagori
Editor: Lin I-hsiu
Illustrator: Natsue Takei
Coordinator: Junko Rodriguez
Formatting: Sota Torigoe

ISBN - 13: 978-0983640240
ISBN - 10: 0983640246

Babel Corporation
Pacific Business News Bldg. #208,
1833 Kalakaua Avenue,
Honolulu, Hawaii 96815

Phone: (808) 946 - 3773
Fax: (808) 946 - 3993

Website: http://www.bookandright.com/

Foreword: Almost All Diseases are Caused by Stress

Throughout my career, I have achieved many new discoveries, especially in the area of my specialty in Immunology. Every time I made a new discovery, I felt as if a new door to the world of life had swung opened.

For example, my most well known discovery was "Regulation of Leukocytes by the Autonomic Nervous System".

This finding revealed that the distribution of leukocytes (immunocytes), which are beneficial to protecting our bodies, are closely regulated by the Autonomic Nervous System (ANS). While I was trying to understand this regulation, I had a revelation.

A simple fact: almost all diseases are caused by stress.

This must sound so simple. Because of its simplicity, many people have missed this fundamental aspect of all biological life. Instead, many researchers unnecessarily thought too much of it and interpreted the causes of diseases as complex, which eventually led to the unfavorable increase in the number of people getting sick.

What I have tried to achieve was to unveil the concept of diseases that had become so complex. I did this by conducting research while focusing on a clue, 'stress'.

Thanks to the clue, I was able to solve so many medical riddles. Consequently, increasing numbers of people are becoming more interested in my understanding of the world of life. I am also happy to hear that people discovered effective tips on living healthier lives or had overcome serious diseases like cancer by reviewing their lifestyles when reading my previous books, which introduced The Abo Immune Theory.

However, over the past several years, I felt that what I had discovered wasn't the whole world of life. I felt that the depth of the world must extend beyond what I have found.

I finally grasped the whole picture of the world of life by following some crucial realizations I had which allowed me to re-examine prior theories.

The results have been concentrated in this book. This is the first book since I published "Your Immune Revolution" which became a bestseller in Japan. I can even say this book was compiled to complete my works.

In this book, unlike my previous works which focused on immunology or the ANS, I have focused on the mechanisms of cells that produce energy for our daily activities.

We have two energy powerhouses in our bodies, within our 60 trillion cells, each of them distinctively different in its characteristics. Human beings use these two powerhouses effectively, depending on various needs. We achieved remarkable evolution by utilizing them. It was in these energy pathways, that the crucial clue to unveiling the causes of human diseases was hidden.

In this book, I have narrowed down the causes of diseases to two roots, and have provided explanations from various angles. These two causes have surfaced by further substantiating what we call stress.

There is no need to think that the causes of diseases are complex. There are only two things we need to be conscious about in order to achieve longevity.

When you understand the meanings of these two things, you will be able to grasp the causes of diseases on your own instead of fully depending on your doctors to find out the causes for you. You will also naturally see your own treatment options. It will also reduce the fear toward cancer.

Our lives are built upon the intricate balance of various activities in our bodies. As you touch the essence of the world of life, you will be moved by it and will experience the excitement of living your life.

You will discover deep meanings of life. Don't you wish to gain the wisdom and utilize it fully in your life? Until now, modern medicine has not offered such a perspective. Instead, it fixated on particular symptoms, and the world of life has not been deeply explored.

I will explain in detail in this book, but humans can finally overcome cancer. The true answer in how to avoid all diseases has been discovered. Therefore, I believe what I explain in my book to be a "once in a hundred years" discovery.

Please take your time to read this book, to transform your awareness and obtain true health by attaining a balanced body and mind.

July 2010

Toru Abo

Table of Contents

The Only Two Causes of All Diseases: Achieve Longevity by Controlling the Hypothermia and Hypoxia!

The Only Two Causes of All Diseases:
Achieve Longevity by Controlling the Hypothermia and Hypoxia!

Chapter 1: Cancer is a "Common Disease"

Cancer is One of the Wisdoms in the Human Body

First of all, let's take a closer look at the essence of all life by first examining the cancers, the disease many people are interested in.

I remember clearly about the day I had a revelation deep inside of me: "cancer is just a common disease". It was on January 10th, 2008.

I will explain later on in detail about what happened on that day, but what I can say now is that this revelation is one of the facts that had surfaced while I was researching on the mechanism of human life.

Modern-day medicine dictates that cancer is a fatal disease. Also, many of you who are reading my book probably consider cancer as a deadly disease and are fearful of it.

In reality, numbers of cancer patients have increased rather than showing any signs of decrease, even though we achieved such advancement in medical technology. According to the Japanese Ministry of Health, Labor and Welfare, 600,000 people have been diagnosed with cancer in Japan every year. Among them, 300,000 die of cancer. Five year survival rate of cancer is 40%, and half of the patients who are diagnosed with cancer would die within five years of the diagnosis.

Also in the U.S., the medical article, Cancer Statistics, 2008 projected a total of 1,437,180 new cases and 565,650 deaths from cancer to occur in the year 2008. The article also mentions that currently one in 4 deaths in the U.S. is due to cancer.

Why has such a common disease as cancer spread out so widely? I have been reporting on the shortcomings of existing cancer treatments that modern medicine offers.

Three major cancer treatments commonly offered by the modern medicine are surgical operation, chemotherapy and radiation therapy. They are known as the three major conventional cancer treatments that are currently available. All these three cancer treatments temporarily suppress the symptoms of cancer. However, they do not remove the "conditions for developing cancer". Unfortunately, because of the nature of modern cancer treatments, many cancer patients will have recurrence in several months or several years after going through the excruciating treatment and removing the cancer.

These conventional treatments can also harm the healthy cells around the cancer cells. As patients face recurrence again and again, they may gradually lose their will to fight cancer. Furthermore, in regards to chemotherapy and radiation therapy, we cannot forget about the side effects caused by these treatments.

Despite these risks, many doctors still cling to the use of the three major conventional cancer treatments. I believe many doctors who use the conventional treatments do not know any other effective treatment methods. They also do not have a full understanding of the fundamental causes of cancer.

Why do humans get cancer? The answer to this question is not so complicated. Follow two factors which cause cancer: stress caused by overworking or concerns from our daily lives, and low body temperature caused by obstruction of blood flow from physical and mental stress. The exposure to stress in addition to the obstruction of blood flow completes the conditions for developing cancer.

I would explain further about these conditions, though, I do not attribute generally known carcinogens as a part of these crucial conditions.

Those carcinogens include eating burnt fish and meat, artificial food additives, smoking, exposure to ultraviolet rays or fungi. They are only triggering factors for developing cancer. Any sensible person will reject the notion that a daily diet of burnt fish and meat alone causes cancer. These are definitely not a main trigger.

Smoking and exposure to ultraviolet rays are often addressed as causes of cancer. However, there are people who are perfectly healthy even though they smoke. Also, if exposures to ultraviolet rays impose such a high risk for developing cancer, then no one will sunbathe any more.

It does not mean these things have no linkage to cancer, but being too sensitive about these triggers does not solve the core problem of developing cancer either. Basically, mentioning these triggering factors to the doctors will not help them at all. As long as doctors focus on the carcinogens, they will fail to pinpoint the direct causes of cancer.

Consequently, the cancer treatments these doctors will construct may only focus on immediate symptoms without looking at the fundamental causes of cancer, which will fail to achieve the complete cure. As a result, patients unknowingly create patterns of recurrence by revisiting the "conditions for cancer development" again.

Do you wish to break away from a cycle of creating the conditions of developing cancer?

If you strongly wish that, then take a close look at the inside of your body instead of focusing on external factors like carcinogens.

One of the mechanisms of human life includes developing cancer. As you read my book, you will realize that the development of cancer is one of the efficient methods the human body uses to respond to difficult body conditions.

This can be said of any other diseases - we need to depart from the idea that cancer is bad. We do not develop diseases because our bodies made a fatal mistake. We get sick because our bodies are methodically responding to the unfavorable conditions of the body. If you gain an understanding of what this means, your perception toward diseases will change dramatically. You will also discover the shortcomings of the three major conventional cancer treatments which focus on removing the cancer cells.

Once you gain these understandings, then you will be able to face cancer more positively, rather than avoiding the treatments because you are afraid of recurrence or side effects.

Cancer is Born in Repetition of Success

"Development of cancer is one of the mechanisms of the human body." – My explanation might have given you some unsettling feelings.

Modern medicine explains that cancer is caused by the mutation of a gene. Its understanding is that the development of cancer is caused by failure and problems within the body. It certainly does not explain it as wisdom of the human body.

Actually, it is true that when a gene that controls the proliferation of genes has a problem, it turns into a cancer gene, which leads to uncontrollable proliferation of the gene itself. Also, the canceration suppressant genes are usually controlling the activities of the cancer gene. When the canceration suppressant genes are disabled, then cancer genes start proliferating uncontrollably, too.

It means that cancer development is triggered either by the activation of the cancer gene or lack of the canceration suppressant gene.

Mutation of a gene commonly exists. However, simply connecting dots by looking at the response of genes does not show us the core causes of the disease, cancer. This misunderstanding happens because all these explanations depart from the idea that cancer is caused by a problem in the human body.

What I discovered and what I would like to let you know is something very different from these ideas. I will gradually guide you through the logic so you will fully understand my discovery. To simply explain it though, what I want to say is: cancer occurs because our bodies follow a logical process to pursue a certain purpose.

It is more correct to say that cancer is not developed by failure in the functions of our body. Rather, it is "born in repetition of success", because if conditions for cancer development exist, then cancer will definitely be developed.

There are logical reasons why a person has cancer. Cancer is not developed because of some problems in your body functions. As we examine the mechanism of development of cancer, the reasons will become very clear to you.

As you read and grasp the concept, you will realize as long as we fully understand the conditions for cancer development, and be conscious about removing such conditions, then spontaneous remission of cancer is possible. Whoever survived cancer -which includes survivors of terminal cancer- followed this process without an exception.

Then what are these conditions for cancer development? My conclusion is that they are hypoxia and hypothermia. **When daily exposure to stress creates hypoxia and hypothermia and such an environment persists, cancer cells may turn up in some body cells.** This is the answer.

Is Disease Evil?

Many people may not immediately grasp the idea that the continuous body environment of hypoxia and hypothermia is a trigger for cancer. I will use examples from the scenes of our daily lives and will explain this in more detail.

In the beginning, I mentioned that cancer is caused by overworking and mental stress in daily life.

Imagine how you feel when you are in stressful situations or emotionally upset. For example, when you work too hard and therefore not sleeping well at night, your face becomes pale and gradually, you become only skin and bones. Naturally, your body temperature becomes lower and the oxygen level in your body decreases as well. Also, when you are emotionally stressed and worried, your blood flows become worse, your face loses its color and your breath grows shallower.

This is what I call the state of hypoxia and hypothermia. If you take a break occasionally and warm up your body, then you can get over this state. However, if you keep yourself busy and do not do anything to alter the condition, then the state of hypoxia and hypothermia becomes your regular state.

You are probably aware that this is not good for our bodies. I would now like to explain reasons why keeping the state of hypoxia and hypothermia eventually leads to the development of cancer.

First, it is important to understand that humans are homoeothermic animals, which means humans require certain temperatures and oxygen levels. If humans lack any of these two elements, then it may make it difficult to live normal daily lives. Consequently, lacking such elements may appear in a loss of facial colors. Then, the human body will try to produce body cells that can adjust to the new environment.

This new cell is the cancer cell. Development of cancer is a result of an adaptive response in which our body cells try to adapt to a new environment of hypoxia and hypothermia.

Getting cancer is no more complicated than this. It is caused by the adaptive response.

It is not necessary to bring up genes to know how cancer is developed. We just need to re-examine how we live every day. Of course, we no longer need to rely on the three conventional cancer treatments. It is possible to cure cancer by changing the lifestyle while being attentive to what caused the hypoxia and hypothermia.

Cancer is caused by a particular lifestyle of people. It is crucial to understand that this is a major premise in understanding the causes of the disease. If we depart from this premise, and start seeking causes of cancer elsewhere -for example in oncogenes or carcinogens- the fundamental answers can get lost.

It will not cure cancer if we remove the cancer cells without re-visiting and re-examining the lifestyle causing our bodies to be in the state of hypoxia and hypothermia. In fact, cancer cells are the cells trying to adapt to the bodily environment of hypoxia and hypothermia.

Cancer is not harmful to our bodies, rather it is a method our bodies use to adapt to a difficult environment. It produces maximum energy efficiency for the body under hypoxia and hypothermia. Cancer is trying to let our body survive. To describe it broadly, your own body is trying to prolong your life by producing the cancer cells.

I hope it is clear to you now what it means then to remove cancer cells.

Cancer is a product of an adaptive response, and it is not a product of failures in our body.

Having this understanding will make a big difference in how you would react emotionally when you are diagnosed with cancer.

Application of this understanding is not limited to cancer, but can be applied to all diseases. We should question the modern medicine's fundamental starting concept that "diseases are evil".

Aerobic, Anaerobic and Cancer

Why then do the body cells turn into cancer cells under the state of hypoxia and hypothermia? I am going to explain this question as the next topic.

I would like to first explain the mechanism of energy production in human cells which is a foundation of biological activities.

Our bodies carry nutrients we obtain from food and oxygen we inhale into our body cells. We convert them into energy for everyday activities. This is how we survive. The reason why humans eat foods and breathe in oxygen is to fuel the energy for the cells in our body, which sums up to 60 trillion cells. Energy production in human cells is fueled by food and oxygen, which is the foundation of biological activities.

The mechanism of energy production can be divided into two processes: the glycolysis pathway and the mitochondrial pathway. To simplify this, it means that humans have two different types of energy powerhouses within human cells.

The glycolysis pathway is a system that converts nutrients from food into energy.

The source of the energy is mainly glucose (carbohydrate), and this system produces energy very quickly due to its simple process of breaking down the glucose. It has an immediate, instantaneous effect, but the amount of energy it can produce is not high.

On the other hand, the mitochondrial pathway system involves many factors including nutrients produced by the glycolysis pathway and oxygen obtained from breathing.

Mitochondria within a cell remove hydrogen (H) from nutrients which is combined with oxygen (O). This process produces massive energy unmatched to the energy produced by the glycolysis pathway.

Animals obtained a ticket to evolution by gaining massive energy through the mitochondrial pathway, but its process is very complicated. When we need to use power immediately, it requires energy produced by the glycolysis pathway as its process is simple and has an instantaneous effect.

In medical terminology, the glycolysis pathway and the mitochondrial pathway is called anaerobic (oxygen independent) and aerobic (oxygen dependent) respectively. We are all living while adapting to the surrounding environment by using these two systems for different purposes. If it is difficult for you to understand, then you can simply consider:

Glycolysis Pathway = Anaerobic Exercise
Mitochondrial Pathway = Aerobic Exercise

For example, the glycolysis pathway (anaerobic exercise), which can produce energy immediately is necessary for quick movements such as short-distance running.

You can try this on your own. When you run at your full speed, you hold your breath, which creates an anaerobic environment. All quick movements involve anaerobic exercise.

Of course, the anaerobic state does not last too long. When we run at our full speed, we quickly become tired and eventually we are unable to move. When glucose is being broken down, substances that make us fatigue are produced such as lactic acid.

Two Energy Powerhouses within Human Cells

	Glycolysis Pathway	Mitochondrial Pathway
Source	Nutrients from Foods (Carbohydrates)	Nutrients from Foods (Carbohydrates, Fat, Protein + Oxygen and Sunlight)
Amount of Energy produced	Small	Massive
Location	Cytoplasm	Mitochondria
Energy Used in	White Muscle, Skin, Sperm	Red Muscle, Brain, Heart, Liver, Ovum
Characteristics	* Instantaneous Force and Divisions * Immediate Reaction * Anaerobic (Oxygen Independent)	* Endurance and Mature * Massive Energy Production * Aerobic (Oxygen Dependent)

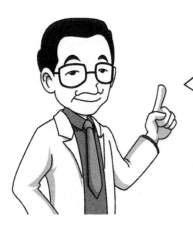

Within human cells that make up our bodies, there exist two distinctive powerhouses; the glycolysis pathway and the mitochondrial pathway. It is very important to utilize both powerhouses in a balanced way.

When we need endurance, we switch to the energy produced in the mitochondrial pathway instead of fueling the energy from the glycolysis pathway. Athletes who are able to exercise for a long period of time are effectively utilizing the energy from the mitochondrial pathway.

Conditions for Cancer Cell Division

To sum up what I explained so far, energy produced by biological activities can be categorized into the following two characteristics:

Glycolysis Pathway = Instantaneous Force
Mitochondrial Pathway = Endurance

Instantaneous force and endurance take turns in accordance with body situations and needs. Also, each pathway has its advantage in different parts of the human body.

For example, for instantaneous activities, we use white muscles (fast muscles). They are consisted of cells without many mitochondria. On the other hand, for activities that require endurance, we use red muscles (slow muscles), which are consisted of cells with many mitochondria.

Muscles full of mitochondria are red, due to the oxygen brought to the mitochondria via iron in the respiratory enzyme.

Iron is naturally white, but when it meets with oxygen, its color turns to red. The reasons why it is often said that aerobic exercise is good for the body is that aerobic exercise activates the energy production in the mitochondria by carrying large amounts of oxygen to red muscles.

However, training only the red muscles does not build a muscular body. To build muscles, cells within the muscles need to be divided rapidly, and these rapid divisions require the anaerobic state.

To build an athletic muscular body, white muscles that do not require oxygen need to be at work. This means energy produced through the glycolysis pathway is necessary. I will explain the detailed mechanisms of it in Chapter 2, but humans' unique characteristic is that we are equipped with two well-balanced muscles: red muscles (endurance = mitochondrial pathway) and white muscles (instantaneous force = glycolysis pathway).

When we understand how our bodies function, the reasons why hypoxia and hypothermia invite canceration of human cells become clarified.

20

The key is the role of the glycolysis pathway. As I mentioned earlier, the glycolysis pathway is a mother ship of instantaneous force, and it is at work during the divisions of cells. Cancer cells also repeat proliferations by cell divisions. The glycolysis pathway becomes advantageous when the state of hypothermia and hypoxia continues in our body.

In short, when the balance of the glycolysis pathway and the mitochondrial pathway is lost, and only the anaerobic glycolysis pathway is being used regularly, then it creates this environment where cancer cells develop easily.

Response to Overcome Emergencies to Your Body

The link between cancer cells and the glycolysis pathway has close connections to the evolution of life.

Actually, not all living beings have mitochondrial pathways which produce massive energy from oxygen.

Only eukaryotes, a group of biological life with a cell nucleus has mitochondria. Prokaryotes such as bacteria lack a cell nucleus and they do not need oxygen. Many prokaryotes proliferate by cell divisions, which means only via the glycolysis pathway.

This means that the canceration is like returning to its ancestors, to prokaryotes. Human cells try to adapt to the environment of hypoxia and hypothermia by utilizing the glycolysis pathway to survive.

I would like to note here that not all use of the glycolysis pathway (cell divisions) lead to the development of cancer. Humans achieved the highest level of evolution, but we also use metabolism by cell divisions just like prokaryotes.

For example, one of the reproductive cells, sperm is activated in the state of hypoxia and hypothermia and proliferates by cell divisions.

That is why the male reproduction organ is an external organ, so that sperm can be cooled to encourage cell divisions. Females' ovum must be warm in order to mature. On the other hand, it is important for males to cool down their reproductive organs partially. If a man wears so much clothing just because it is very cold outside, his body is too warm and may prevent cell divisions of sperms.

I derail from the main topic here, but I want to make a point that the recent issue of men's sperm decrease may be caused by the lifestyle of men who stay in a warm room and do not cool down the area between their legs. Decreased sperm count is not only caused by the endocrine disrupters such as dioxin.

Also, skin cells have a tendency for cell divisions. When we go through the winter barefooted at home, the skin on the soles of our feet becomes thicker. This is a result of cell divisions encouraged by the cool temperature. On the other hand, if you keep the sole of your feet warm, then the skin gets softer.

Actually, I have also tried it myself. If you put a hot water bottle against your skin, you will see your skin become thinner and see veins appear through the skin.

This happens because warm body temperatures activate the mitochondrial pathway, and this condition discourages cell divisions.

This shows that canceration can be suppressed by warming our body. Some parts of the human body function better in lower temperatures, but overall, if our body temperatures stay down, then it creates perfect conditions for the development of cancer.

Imagine yourself in freezing cold weather in the winter. Being cold means creating hypothermia, creating a stressful situation for the body.

Also, imagine that you're running away from an enemy. Your face turns pale. Or, imagine attacking your enemy. Your breathing becomes shallow, and naturally you'll be in the state of hypoxia. Also, adrenalin is secreted which lead to hyperglycemia.

Having hypothermia and hypoxia, or hyperglycemia and high blood pressure (hypertension) can impose stress on the human body. These conditions can cause diseases. I will explain how hyperglycemia and hypertension stress our bodies later in this book.

All these body reactions, however, is a response to emergencies that are occurring in our bodies and it should be regarded as an adaptive response. If you follow this logic, then you can understand that disease does not come from failure of body functions.

In reality, when I observe cancer cells through the microscope, I can see them diligently dividing cells. When I look at cancer cell without preconceptions about them, they do not look like evil cells. Instead, they look like the cells which have pure souls.

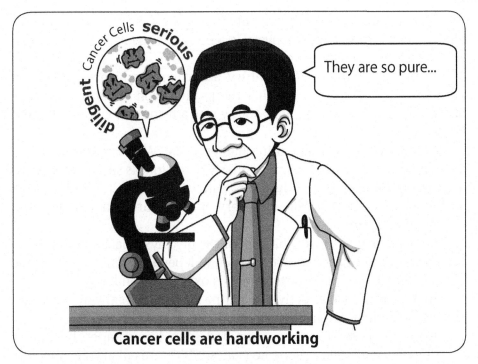

Cancer cells are hardworking

Having cancer is a result of our bodies responding normally to stress. But if we continue to let our bodies be exposed to stress by constantly overworking and not resolving things that upset us emotionally, then our bodies will be stuck in the world of the glycolysis pathway. At the end, our bodies will give up.

This perfectly depicts the old saying; "more than enough is too much". How you perceive the development of cancer can change everything. Whether we look at the canceration as a failure in our body functions or as a normal adaptive response of our bodies, change each person's choice of treatment methods and choice of lifestyles.

I would like to repeat that cancer develops in ordinary daily lives. Modern medicine failed to understand cancer by complicating the interpretation of the disease and consequently made cancer an incurable disease.

A Huge Clue Hidden in the Research from 80 Years Ago

You probably understand now that the mechanism of the development of cancer is closely linked to the energy production mechanism within human cells.

It is my discovery finding the linkage between stress and hypothermia and hypoxia, but my discovery is a product achieved by following a lot of research done by my predecessors.

In the beginning of 20th century, a German biochemist, Otto Warburg (1883 - 1970), indicated that the proliferation of cancer cells are observed, when the glycolysis pathway was advantageous in the human body.

Details will be explained in chapter 7, but Warburg is one of the most important biochemists, particularly noted for his success in revealing the mechanism of the glycolysis pathway. He won the Nobel Prize in Physiology of 1931 for his discovery of the nature and action of "the respiratory enzyme".

Remember that the mechanism of the glycolysis pathway that Warburg discovered was anaerobic (oxygen independent), contrary to aerobic (the mitochondrial pathway which is oxygen dependent).

In Warburg's time, activities of the glycolysis pathway were described as "fermentation".

In the process of making wine and sake, fermentation begins by shutting off the oxygen to activate yeasts, which are eukaryotic microorganisms. By creating the anaerobic environment, it encourages glycolysis, which means the activation of the glycolysis pathway encourages the alcohol fermentation.

You might have realized now, but cancer cell divisions and proliferations are promoted under similar conditions of alcohol fermentation. Hypothermia and hypoxia are perfect conditions for the proliferation of cancer.

Cancer cells have very small amount of mitochondria despite the large size of the cell. **Cancer cells proliferate without using the mitochondrial pathway (oxygen).**

Warburg's vision in focusing on cancer cells proliferated by using the glycolysis pathway was an excellent foresight. His idea is called the "Warburg Effect", and even after his death, his research was inherited by many who followed him in different research projects. However, it is far from stating that the truth about cancer was discovered by those who followed him.

One reason for that is -as I mentioned earlier- as genetic analysis technology advanced, the idea of cancer being caused by genetic mutation became widely accepted. As a result, looking at the fundamentals of the "conditions for the development of cancer" was lost.

Also, drugs such as the ones used for chemotherapy became major treatment options over the course of many years. Fundamental questions of the Warburg effect was lost and forgotten in those times.

I say that if researchers do not see beyond the preconception of viewing cancer cells as failures of the human body, Warburg's research will not be fully utilized. Also, the reality of people suffering from cancer cells that proliferate under the state of hypothermia and hypoxia will not change without realizing this preconception.

I would like to bring up once again that cancer proliferation occurs when conditions of hypothermia and hypoxia exist and the glycolysis pathway is dominant in energy productions. If we shift our attention to these conditions, we discover the heart of the disease called cancer.

Spontaneous Remission of Cancer Often Occurs

To sum up what I explained so far, cancer can effectively survive in the world of glycolysis pathways which encourages cell divisions.

Again, development of cancer is not caused by failed functions in the human body, but by the normal adaptive response of the human body. When we understand what this means, then we can further explore how we can encourage spontaneous remission of cancer cells and stop the multiplication of those cells.

In my opinion, **retracting the cancer cells is not so difficult. We need to change the body environment to an environment where cancer cells cannot thrive, by changing the state of hypothermia and hypoxia to the environment in which the mitochondrial pathway can be dominant.**

There are many clinical case examples in which spontaneous remission of cancer have been reported. Many of these cases do not involve the three conventional cancer treatments, but it can be found in the treatments done by utilizing alternative medicine.

An example of alternative therapy includes Immunotherapy via the Autonomic Nervous System (ANS), which helps to promote the immune system in the body. A common factor in successful alternative medicine is that all successful therapies involve with "keeping the patients' bodies warm".

Perfect foundations for cell divisions are consisted of hypothermia and hypoxia. It is self-evident that if we provide the opposite kind of environment for cancer cells, they cannot live in it. Keeping our bodies warm does not only promote effectiveness of immune cells, but it can also remove the comfortable body environment for cancer cells to thrive because it will shrink the glycolysis pathway.

Modern medicine encourages the removal of cancer cells by implementing early discovery and early treatment of cancer. Their starting point of the diagnosis is that cancer is a failure. In this direction, the modern medicine technology and research were polished and advanced in recent years.

However, early discovery of cancer does not necessarily prevent development of cancer entirely. We don't feel it, but canceration occurs almost on daily basis inside of our bodies. It is not so special thing.

Removing a small cancer cell is not a perfect solution. Even if it was not removed, many cases are reported that spontaneous remission of cancer occurred. The number of cancer patients will not change by recommending cancer screenings anyway.

If you are worried about getting cancer, then you should first re-examine your own lifestyle. Modify your lifestyle if you live your life in a flat-out dash speed like the one which embodies the glycolysis pathway and anaerobic exercise. Change to a slower lifestyle, which utilizes the mitochondrial pathway and aerobic exercise.

Specific examples are, keeping your body warm and maintaining a slower breathing. A lifestyle that is advantageous to the mitochondrial pathway will reduce stress, and eventually it will remove the conditions that can develop into cancer.

Reasons Why a Serious Person Gets Cancer

A lifestyle that relies on the glycolysis pathway is in other words, a stressful life.

That is how stress has a strong connection to cancer. If you wish to understand the essence of cancer, please understand this point.

In principle, we live by maintaining the balance in using the two energy pathways, the glycolysis pathway and the mitochondrial pathway.

If we use the glycolysis pathway too much, then the body becomes fatigue due to the accumulation of lactic acid created by the lack of oxygen intake. When this happens, we can recover by taking a relaxing break which changes the energy source to the mitochondrial pathway.

Also, when you have something that upsets you emotionally, your body becomes stressed and fall into the state of hypothermia and hypoxia.

It is a natural process to have some issues keeping you in deep thoughts, but many will reset their thoughts once realizing that thinking over and over again do not solve the fundamental problem. When this realization for change comes, people usually can depart from the glycolysis pathway controlling their body environment.

However, many people who are serious about everything cannot let go of their worrisome thoughts. Also, some people can be totally absorbed in one thing, and consequently let their bodies be exposed to the conditions of hypothermia and hypoxia for a long period of time.

By overworking, not sleeping enough and constantly losing ourselves in worrisome thoughts, we place burden on our bodies. Our bodies remarkably always try to adapt to such negative conditions.

Body cells become cancer cells to adapt to these unbalanced and stressful lifestyles by supporting the activation of the glycolysis pathway.

In a way, we can say that our bodies try to maintain the balance by turning body cells into cancer.

This is the true meaning of maintaining the balance in our body. When we understand this, then we can also see that the cancer cells do not necessarily keep proliferating. By changing our internal environment to the one advantageous to mitochondrial pathways, we will have a possibility of encouraging the spontaneous remission of cancer. In reality, there are many people who survived terminal cancer.

You may now understand that the cancer is not something you need to be fearful of. Cancer is developed, because body cells follow the relation of cause and effect. Development of cancer is closely affected by our lifestyle.

When people hear the word 'cancer', many people may feel terrified. There is no reason for that. What we need to be afraid of, is by being terrified like that, the cancer cells may proliferate.

For example, when you go for a cancer screening, your feeling may constantly alternate between hope and fear, needing to face worrisome thoughts. It can be said that by suggesting the cancer screening, doctors are causing more stress to patients, which may affect the patients in developing cancer cells.

Same thing can be said about annual physical examinations. I believe it is not always necessary for you to continue going to these medical examinations, especially when it frightens you.

I, myself, have barely gone to these medical examinations and screening since I established the ANS theory and understood the mechanism of diseases.

To begin with, there are better things we should be mindful of in our daily lives, rather than spending time going to these examinations and screenings. You should not think that everything will be fine just because you go to the screening or medical examinations regularly. We should be mindful of living a balanced lifestyle, and that is what's important.

Stress itself is not a bad thing. I am also not saying not to ever pull overtimes at work. It is best to find moderate ground in finding balance in your life without deciding your lifestyle in black and white polarization.

The important thing is to determine which lifestyle you would like to live: whether you want to live in an unstable health condition which can develop cancer or to live a more comfortable and balanced lifestyle for your body and soul.

If you cannot visualize the meaning of a balanced lifestyle yet, I hope you will take some tips from this book.

What I've written in this book are all scientific facts which were revealed by studying biological activities. Please open your mind and absorb the wisdom of life, and practice the tips in this book in your daily life. You will gradually understand what it means to have a balanced lifestyle.

Cancer is Caused by an Ineffective Lifestyle

Even though we understand the importance of a balanced lifestyle, only a few people can actually practice it in reality. Some of you might already have cancer, because your body relied on the glycolysis pathway for a long time which resulted in creating an unbalanced environment within your own body.

Once developed, it takes time to cure cancer entirely. Having cancer shows the results of how you have lived your life so far. There is no need for you to panic, but receive the news as a good opportunity to re-examine your lifestyle.

Having cancer may mean that you have already lived a productive life packed with experiences. You worked extra hard which forced you to use the glycolysis pathway. Some people who died of cancer at a very young age, may have lived a full life unique to that person in return of living an unbalanced lifestyle.

I believe it is one way to regard terminal cancer as god-send and let it be, when people find out the diagnosis late due to the delay in discovery. Often times, modern medicine's excruciating treatments only leave the patients with unnecessary pains and sufferings.

If you rather not think that terminal cancer as god-send, then please study the characteristics of cancer that I explained so far, and make up your mind and try to depart from your current lifestyle of hypothermia and hypoxia – this is the shortcut for a cure.

Not all advanced cancers result in death, and many examples of miraculous recoveries have been reported.

I suggest for cancer patients to try all treatment methods that are known for being effective for cancer without believing that the major cancer treatments available today are the only solutions for the cure. In addition to choosing cancer treatment methods, re-visit your own life. There will be many things you may want to re-adjust, such as lifestyles and ways of thinking.

In the other words, people who have cancer are the people who are not effectively using the mitochondrial pathway which can produce massive energy for them. That way of living is very ineffective which is against the evolution of life.

As I explained earlier, living beings achieved remarkable evolution by obtaining the mitochondrial pathway which allowed for aerobic activities.

It is only natural to develop cancer when we live a daily life by hardly breathing. We are not making full use of the ability of the mitochondrial pathway then, but using full capacity of the glycolysis pathway, which is only good for producing instantaneous force.

If you lead your life now by only using the glycolysis pathway at full force, then please know there is a slower lifestyle you can live in, the one which encourages the mitochondrial pathway. Knowing it is a starting point and knowing there is an alternative way of living may become a turning point in your life.

Breathing Exercise that Can Change Your Life

To make the mitochondrial pathway advantageous, it is very important to inhale a lot of oxygen into your body by practicing deep breathing. I would like to refer to the important role of oxygen at the end of this chapter.

When you get sick, you would breathe heavily, which shows that the body is requiring you to breathe in more because your body is in a state of hypoxia.

Same thing can be said when you get angry and irritated. When you lose your temper, your breath becomes shallow or you may hold your breath. If the irritating situation continues, then the hypoxia becomes chronic.

With shallow breathing, obviously, not all body cells are getting enough oxygen. In this environment, the mitochondria pathway will not be switched on due to the lack of oxygen.

As a consequence, the glycolysis pathway dominates energy production, which will result in a prolonged state of hypothermia and hypoxia, creating perfect conditions for the development of cancer.

When you know these mechanisms within your body, you will realize deep breathing is a way to maintain the balance of your body and mind.

Since the old days, high monks practiced Zen meditation using abdominal breathing. The deep breathing helped to calm down anger, irritations and bewilderments, while allowing the glycolysis pathway to rest. It was the wisdom of shifting the body to the mitochondria pathway and to the world of enlightenment.

I also believe that aerobic exercises, such as Tai Chi and Yoga have been cherished for many years for the same reasons.

In addition to keeping your body warm, be mindful about replenishing your body with fresh oxygen through moderate exercises – this is the best way to restore your energy and to free yourself from a stressful daily life that can easily lean toward a life trapped in the glycolysis pathway.

It is important to practice these things in your daily life. Take a break effectively. It will lead to the prevention of cancer.

I would like to mention an additional story here. Numbers of erythrocyte and hemoglobin -both of which are carriers of oxygen to cells- increase when exercising at the places where oxygen level is low, such as at high altitudes on a mountain. This happens because the body adapts to the environment of low oxygen and cell divisions in bone marrow are promoted.

The human body tries to adapt to the environment of low oxygen by increasing the volume of oxygen carried to the cells. If the person is not properly trained, there is a risk of getting altitude sickness. However, when the training is successful, once the trained person returns to the lower ground, the mitochondrial pathway will be able to produce energy more efficiently due to the development of high oxygen replenishment rate. Marathon runners use this training method to increase their endurance.

Shortly before the 2010 World Cup Soccer, Team Japan had a training camp in Switzerland located at a high altitude. As you all know, Team Japan had a great record in the 2010 World Cup.

Recently, using a machine called an oxygen capsule is becoming popular as a way to resolve oxygen deficiency as well.

By using this machine, it is possible to inhale oxygen artificially, which activates the mitochondrial pathway in a short period of time. This allows the human body to recover from fatigue and tiredness quickly, but I believe it is more important to physically take a good rest to recover from fatigue and tiredness.

For professional athletes who consume large amounts of energy constantly may have good merit from using this machine. However, relying heavily on machinery means to "live your life too quickly".

There is a very fine line between growth and aging. I believe it is

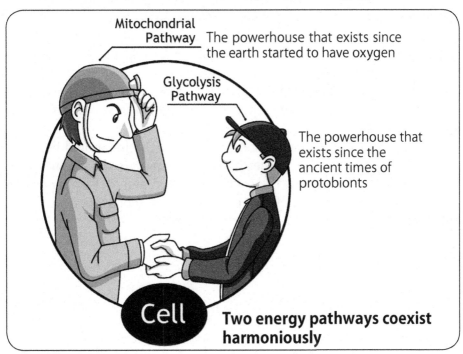

Mitochondrial Pathway The powerhouse that exists since the earth started to have oxygen

Glycolysis Pathway

The powerhouse that exists since the ancient times of protobionts

Cell **Two energy pathways coexist harmoniously**

more natural to practice breathing exercises and aerobic exercises in everyday life at our own paces.

At any rate, we all need to breathe to live.

Within our bodies, two energy pathways co-exist: the mitochondrial pathway which requires a lot of oxygen, and the glycolysis pathway which dislikes oxygen and only uses nutrients from foods.

In the next chapter, we will take a closer look at the origin of mitochondria which holds a crucial key to maintaining biological life. Let's examine further about the mysterious linkage between the glycolysis pathway and mitochondrial pathway. It will give you a clue for living a balanced life which can prevent cancer.

From Abo Laboratory 1:
Disease is Not Caused by the Body's Failure

In this chapter, I explained the most important point in this book: "Cancer develops as a result of a normal adaptive response of the body, reacting to the state of hypoxia and hypothermia". When we all understand that cancer is not born because of a failed function of the body as the modern medicine has portrayed, perceptions toward the conventional cancer treatments may change dramatically.

Diseases, in essence, are a kind of common biological responses (adaptive responses) to an emergency which is triggered by the daily stress that we are exposed to due to overworking and emotional distress. You will be convinced that "Oh, it was after all this simple," after understanding this adaptive response as is and not to complicate it further.

In terms of treatment methods, the starting point should be to escape from hypoxia and hypothermia. Simple answers of "keeping your body warm", "cutting down the overtime hours" and "breathing deeply and slowly" will appear as effective treatment methods when we follow this starting point.

Chapter 2: Two Mechanisms that Mobilize Life

Mitochondria's Ancestor is Bacteria

In the last chapter, I explained that we have two energy powerhouses within a human cell; the mitochondrial pathway and the glycolysis pathway.

The glycolysis pathway produces energy only from nutrients (carbohydrates) while the mitochondrial pathway produces energy by combining oxygen that we breathe in with the nutrients. The mitochondrial pathways can use fat and protein as an energy source in addition to carbohydrates (sugar).

When an element of the mitochondrial pathways is added to the cell, it dramatically increases the energy production capacity of the cell. However, this does not mean that the glycolysis pathway is unnecessary. These two distinctive powerhouses coexist within the 60 trillion cells in our bodies, delegating specific roles to maintain life.

Why do we have to have two powerhouses then?

Actually, this question is a crucial one to fully understand the very reason why humans get diseases and suffer from illnesses like cancer.

The mechanism of biological energy production is very complex, and each process plays a specific role within the complex mechanism. Also, each has its own history of how they came to play that role. In this history, a secret clue of all diseases is hidden.

We humans originate from a single cell, unicellular organism. Over the course of billions of years, it has achieved a remarkable evolution by adapting to the environment on earth. It has turned into a multicellular organism by equipping itself with an energy powerhouse, mitochondria. It soon developed tissues and organs, and had increased in size.

Let's take a look at the history of living organisms by starting at the beginning when life began.

It is said to be about 3.8 billion years ago when there was no oxygen in the atmosphere. Atmosphere on the earth at that time mainly consisted of gaseous nitrogen and carbon dioxide. Apparently, living organisms had to live by utilizing the energy produced by the glycolysis pathway.

In the beginning, protobionts proliferated through cell divisions in the anaerobic world. It can be said that they lived in the 'immortal environment'.

When they lacked nutrition or are exposed to a harsh environment, these organisms stop their living functions. However, they can be reactivated when all conditions for their survival are met again. It is a characteristic of such living organisms to live forever as long as the organisms do not lose their bodies; for example by getting burned.

It was approximately 2 billion years ago when a dramatic change arrived to this immortal world of protobionts. Some of the ancient living organisms (prokaryote) became photosynthetic organisms, which started to convert sunlight into energy. And these organisms began to thrive.

Photosynthesis is a system of converting water and carbon dioxide into nutrients (carbohydrate) while utilizing energy from sunlight. This process of conversion releases oxygen. As photosynthetic organisms thrived, oxygen was released to the atmosphere that predominantly consisted of nitrogen and carbon dioxide gas. It led to a gradual increase in the level of oxygen concentration in the atmosphere.

At the time, protobionts survived comfortably in the world of the glycolysis pathway. Increase in the level of oxygen concentration was threatening their lives.

Currently, oxygen occupies 21% of the atmosphere. By 2 billion years ago, oxygen concentration levels had increased to around 2%. Anaerobic bacteria living at that time faced a life-threatening crisis just by having the oxygen concentration level increase from 0% to 2%.

During this crisis, organisms that could effectively produce energy from oxygen had appeared. Actually, these aerobic bacteria (bacteria which utilized oxygen) are considered to be the ancestors of mitochondria, a tiny organ in our body.

Reasons Why Bacteria Turned into an Energy Powerhouse

You might be surprised by my explanation; an energy powerhouse within our body cell was a kind of bacterium, when we explore its origin.

However, it is considered that our human cells originated from a bacterium equipped with the mitochondrial pathway, which evolved by mitochondria starting to live on a unicellular organism that was surviving solely on the glycolysis pathway. Consequently, these organisms began to evolve rapidly by being able to obtain massive amounts of energy.

So, how did the ability to convert oxygen to energy lead to evolution? I will explain the answer to this question later on, but first, I would like to explain the reasons why aerobic bacteria started to live on anaerobic bacteria.

Let's picture this: locations where aerobic bacteria became active, oxygen are being consumed, creating a partial area with no oxygen.

Perhaps, some of the ancient organisms living only on the glycolysis pathway (anaerobic bacteria) fled to an area with no oxygen in order to survive. Anaerobic bacteria had to base their survival on the aerobic bacteria, which consumed oxygen for them. On the other hand, it was a chance for aerobic bacteria since they could utilize the nutrients (lactic acid) that anaerobic bacteria produced via the glycolysis pathway.

I established a scenario: Because one could benefit from the other, aerobic bacteria and anaerobic bacteria gradually gathered together. Some of them fused cell membranes and as time went on, they achieved unification while the progenitor cells (anaerobic bacteria) absorbed the aerobic bacteria.

When we look at this from the perspective of mitochondria, it was parasitism. However, from the perspective of the progenitor cells, we can say it was a union.

This way, the mitochondria could also feed on a part of the carbohydrates produced by the glycolysis pathway and a balanced co-existence was made possible.

Of course, the aerobic bacteria (mitochondria) that became parasites were independent living organisms to begin with, so it carried its own genes (DNA).

However, after the mitochondria started to live on its host, it gave parts of its DNA to the host. This prevented the mitochondria to live on independently. This is how aerobic bacteria turned into mitochondria, a tiny organelle within the human body.

Because of its origin and history, mitochondria carry its own DNA even though it is an organelle within parts of the human cell. However, it uses the DNA only when it needs to for its own division and copying, while it relies on the host's DNA for any other functions.

Mitochondria that produces massive energy

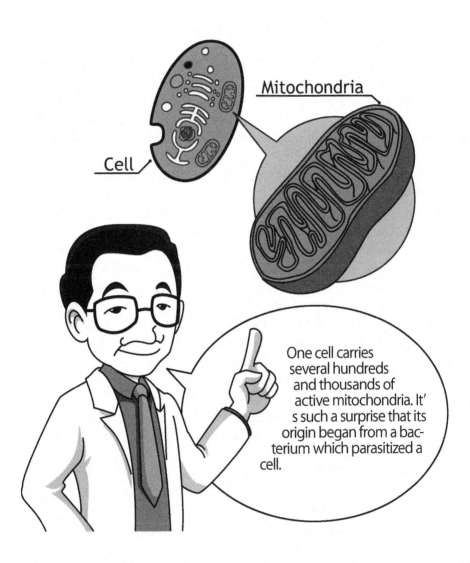

Oxygen Produces Massive Energy

Anyway, the symbiosis between two living beings (union of two cells) I mentioned in the previous chapter happened about 2 billion years ago.

Of course, it was not easy for them to stay together in the beginning, as one liked oxygen and the other disliked oxygen. Their marriage was unstable for about 8 hundred million years, on and off. Finally after that, they achieved a perfect union.

The result of the perfect union was the creation of a cell which became the prototype of the human cell. It was equipped with various organelles, such as a cell nucleus which stored DNA, in addition to mitochondria that parasitized.

The bacterium before the mitochondria parasitized cell was a prokaryote. A newly married cell is a eukaryote.

About 1.2 billion years ago, a stable eukaryote, our direct ancestor was born after overcoming various obstacles.

Around this time, the cell started to have the ability to multicellularize as well. Now you can see how a perfect union of cells in the ancient time remains within our 60 trillion cells, and why we have two different energy powerhouses within the cells.

Until a cell carried mitochondria, it was repeating cell divisions in the world of the glycolysis pathway. However, when it started to carry mitochondria, it entered the world of 'complication'.

Complication, because calls started to leave offspring by going through the process of growth, change and death.

On the other hand, bacteria which did not achieve the union still live in the immortal world as one of prokaryote while repeating cell divisions.

Our human cells also go through cell divisions. However, as I mentioned earlier, it is not unlimited. Also in our cells, leftover nutrients from the glycolysis pathway are passed onto the mitochondrial pathway which utilized them for producing massive amounts of energy.

To better understand such a relationship, I will go through the overview of the energy production mechanism in human cells, which consisted of two pathways as you already know.

When we eat foods, nutrients contained in the foods will be absorbed by the intestine, and it is carried further via blood and lymph fluid to the cells in the whole body. The nutrient converted into the energy within a cell is mainly carbohydrates (glucose).

Energy for our daily activities is produced in the process as nutrients contained in rice, bread and potatoes are being broken down.

This is how the glycolysis pathway produces energy from carbohydrate. However, the energy produced by the glycolysis pathway is not enough to sustain life. As I explained in Chapter 1, it is produced instantly and consumed instantly. It can only produce enough energy to maintain the instantaneous force of daily activities of humans.

Of course, supplemental energy needs to be created from somewhere else. This is where the energy powerhouse within the mitochondrial pathway comes in.

Nutrients being resolved within the glycolysis pathway are further resolved inside of mitochondria, which produce hydrogen. When this hydrogen is combined with oxygen which is brought in via a different pathway, a massive amount of energy for our daily activities is produced.

One glucose molecule is converted to 2 molecules of energy produced by the glycolysis pathway. The mitochondrial pathway on the other hand, produces 36 molecules of energies. You can see how large the amount of energy the mitochondrial pathway produces.

Energy produced by the mitochondrial pathway does not have instantaneous force similar to the energy produced by the glycolysis pathway. However, by utilizing the massive energy created by hydrogen, it maintains the daily activities and life of large animals, such as humans.

Energy Production Mechanism within Human Cells

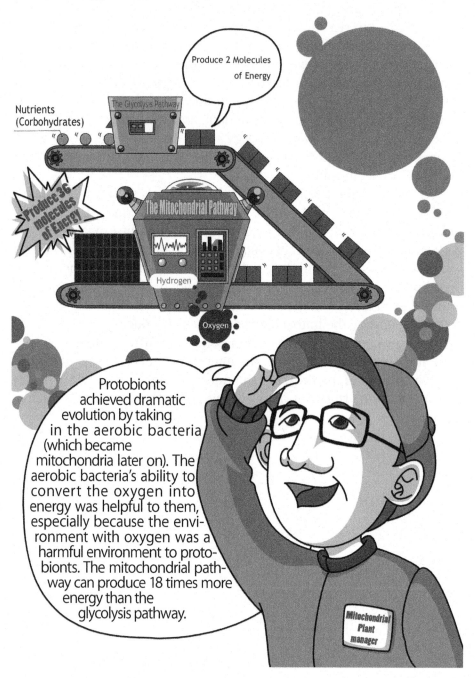

Why are There White Muscles and Red Muscles?

So far, we looked at the origin of mitochondria and the mechanism behind energy productions. I would like you to understand that it is not correct to think each cell only contains a single mitochondrion.

It depends on which parts of the body we are looking at. However, it is understood that there are some hundreds to thousands of mitochondria scattered within one cell. It is as if many power plants are in operation converting raw materials of oxygen into energy. As a whole, it fuels our body in order to maintain the daily activities of humans.

Which part of the body contains the most mitochondria? Easy ones to list here are; a part of the skeletal muscle (red muscle), the brain, nerves and the liver.

Among the red muscle, the skeletal muscle (also known as the inner muscle because it is located inside of the muscle) is said to especially contain five thousand mitochondria within a cell. Also, four thousand mitochondria within the brain and nerve cells and two thousands within liver cells were also observed.

Furthermore, a matured ovum contains one hundred thousand mitochondria within a cell (Details will be explained in Chapter 5).

All these parts of the body have characteristics of rarely going through cell divisions, since the mitochondrial pathway is working more dominantly in all these cells. For example, cell divisions in brains and nerves stop at the end of childhood. After that, it solidifies and works as is for a lifetime, like the saying "Give me a child for the first seven years, and you may do what you want with him afterwards". There is also an old similar proverb in Japan, "A three year old's soul lasts until the child becomes one hundred years old". Perhaps this reflects the characteristic of mitochondria.

The common ground for all these tissues and organs that I mentioned is that they all require massive amounts of oxygen to activate the mitochondria.

In the previous chapter, I mentioned that the muscle cells which contain many mitochondria are colored red. The iron within the respiratory enzyme is being oxidized by the large amount of oxygen brought in, which turns its color to red. Same thing can be said for the brain and liver.

Let's organize our understandings so far with the following:

Many mitochondria in cells → Muscles turn red = Red muscle
A few mitochondria in cells → Muscles do not turn red = White muscle

As I mentioned earlier, white muscles are muscles which exist near the surface of the body, in contrast to the inner muscle (red muscles) which exist inside of the body. White muscles are used when we carry heavy things or when we jump.

It should ring a bell when **we say that white muscles producing instantaneous force depend on the glycolysis pathway, and red muscles producing endurance depend on the mitochondrial pathway. Red muscle is also called the 'slow muscle' and the white muscle is called the 'fast muscle'. These distinctions come from the difference in energy pathways that the muscle cell utilizes.**

I will give you an easy example. In track-and-field sports, short-distance running require white muscle (the glycolysis pathway). On the other hand, long-distance running such as during marathons uses red muscle (the mitochondrial pathway). It is also the same reason why a flounder which hides along the ocean floor to catch its prey with instant movement is a white fish, while a tuna fish which swims thousands of kilometers for migration is a red fish.

Usain Bolt, the short-distance sprinter, who set new world records repeatedly at the 2008 Beijing Olympics, effectively uses white muscles that are equipped with the glycolysis pathway to fully utilize the powerful instantaneous force. The world of the glycolysis pathway is anaerobic, so if a sprinter breathes even a little bit during a run, the glycolysis pathway (white muscles) is restrained. Thus he/she becomes unable to create such a powerful instantaneous force.

Of course, the energy produced by the glycolysis pathway does not last long and the amount of energy produced by the pathway is small. The maximum distance for the short track running is 400 meters, and the world record is 43 seconds for men and 47 seconds for women. Humans can hold their breath for about 1 minute, so we can conclude that this time is an estimate of the limit of how long the glycolysis pathway can last.

Because of this limit for the glycolysis pathway, longer distance requires more energy and the body switches to aerobic exercises via the mitochondrial pathway. At the end of this spectrum, there is a marathon in which people complete a 42.195 kilometres (26.2 miles) run.

In many sports, athletes compete between winning or losing while the body switches its energy production between the glycolysis pathway and the mitochondrial pathway.

What Happens if You Train in an Anaerobic Environment?

Let's think more about the relationship between muscle and energy pathways.

In the world of sports, athletes have been utilizing the unique characteristics of two energy pathways in various ways.

For example, interval running and occlusion training effectively use attributes of the glycolysis pathway.

Interval running is a training method where runners run while alternating between running fast and running slow, one after another, which strengthens instantaneous force. By repeating running fast and slow, the instantaneous force of the glycolysis pathway is being strengthened. Professional athletes use this training method, but we can all utilize this training to strengthen the balance of both instantaneous force and endurance. For example, we can alternate between walking fast and slow when you take a walk outside.

Occlusion training applies occlusion to limit the amount of blood going through the veins by wearing specialized straps on the target parts of the body during training to effectively build muscle.

When we limit the amount of blood going through the vein, it creates an anaerobic environment. It strengthens activities in the glycolysis pathway. Also, cell generation as well as cell division is encouraged. As a result, in a short period of time and without much stress, people can achieve better results in muscle building than working out in a regular environment.

By using these training methods, it is possible to activate two energy pathways. However, there is a limit. Actually, our bodies have a tendency to rely on the mitochondrial pathway more as we age.

Many sports athletes retire at age 30. I think it is because as we age, it becomes more difficult to utilize the glycolysis pathway or instantaneous force.

On the other hand, seniors can play sports well, like golf and archery which only require slower body movements. Playing golf only requires the glycolysis pathway when we take a shot. As long as golfers effectively utilize the mitochondrial pathway, they can play golf comfortably and effectively even at an old age.

Also, Budou or martial arts in the East includes Aikido (Japanese art of weaponless self-defense), Qi-Gong (Chinese exercise, meditation and medicine) and Tai Chi (traditional Chinese shadow boxing), which can all be practiced regardless of age. All these exercises share a common concept of not including fast body movements and placing importance on breathing exercises (oxygen supplementation).

Aerobic exercise activates the mitochondrial pathway, strengthening endurance and activating cells within our body. It has health benefits as well. Masters of Budou and martial arts are also masters of utilizing the mitochondrial pathway effectively.

Secrets of the Swimsuit Mass-Produced World Records

I would like to talk a little more about sports-related topics to further illustrate the relationship between the glycolysis pathway and the mitochondrial pathway.

At the Beijing Olympic I just mentioned, swimmers who wore swimsuits called the LZR Racer Suit broke many world records at the swimming events.

The LZR Racer Suit was developed in association with organizations such as NASA (The National Aeronautics and Space Administration). Its seams are ultrasonically welded for better repellent of water which reduces drag to its limit. It compresses the body, reducing the uneven shape of the human body to further reduce drag. It is said that when swimmers wear this swimsuit, they can swim in the water very smoothly.

All the readers who went through the previous chapters might have found more advantages of the LZR Racer Suit, other than the reduction of drag. However, the swimsuit manufacturer was not aware of the other advantages. I was able to confirm this because I wrote to the company about what I will explain below. They replied to me that they did not intend for the suit to have such benefits.

When swimmers wear highly compressed swimsuits which require assistance by other person to pull them on, it limits the amount of blood going through the veins. Consequently, the whole body becomes low in oxygen. This is as the same mechanism as in the Occlusion training. It skyrockets the energy released by the glycolysis pathway, enabling the body to achieve strong instantaneous force. World records can be broken as a result of this.

Swimming is a sport where the glycolysis pathway is advantageous, because swimmers hold their breath under the water. When the amount of blood flowing through the veins is limited while the breath is held, it creates a synergistic effect increasing instantaneous force further.

I would not call it proof, but when we look at swimmers who wear the LZR Racer Suit for longer distance swimming events - longer than 100 meters - they cannot break world records that easily. I think this is because long distance swimming requires some energy production through the mitochondrial pathway as well, and they cannot only rely on the energy produced through the glycolysis pathway for these events.

Actually, even before the introduction of the LZR Racer Suit, attempts to achieve better records by utilizing the anaerobic environment caught some attentions in the news.

For example, a Japanese backstroke swimmer, Daichi Suzuki, implemented a 'Vassallo kicks' swimming style in which he swam the first 30 meters underwater and won the gold medal at the 1988 Summer Olympics in Seoul. After a while, 'Vassallo kicks' was limited to the first 15 meters. By submerging underwater for a longer period of time, he forcefully created an anaerobic environment and strengthened the glycolysis pathway (instantaneous force). That was a secret of his effective instantaneous force.

Another swimmer, Shigehiro Takahashi of Chukyo University who was considered a medal contender for the breaststroke events at one point, did not qualify for the Moscow Olympics because his swimming style was considered against the rules. His head was completely submerged underwater during the race. After his disqualification, the rule was changed allowing for his style. He then qualified for the Los Angeles and Seoul Olympics consecutively. The merit of this swimming style also has close relationship with creating an anaerobic environment which results in the activation of the glycolysis pathway.

The glycolysis pathway and the mitochondrial pathway are two unique characteristics and abilities of human beings. By using each pathway's ability effectively, we can better control instantaneous force and endurance. When athletes grasp that fine line of control, they will be able to maximize their abilities to compete.

Live Long in the World of Aerobic

I have just mentioned that by using the glycolysis pathway effectively, athletes can create an anaerobic environment to strengthen the instantaneous force – this situation is not unique to athletes, but apply to all of us.

In our daily lives, this can be most apparent when we become angry. Imagine when you have bursts of anger. You are naturally holding your breath when you get angry. When we continue to hold our breath, the amount of blood flow into the veins will be limited. This will lead to hypothermia.

I have explained that hypothermia and hypoxia are the conditions of development of cancer, so you might think, "I knew getting angry is not good for my health!"

However, the state of hypoxia does not last too long. It is like a holding your own breath. After about one minute, it will switch to the aerobic state.

This is how anger naturally recedes. We don't usually need to worry about getting angry being bad for our health, because our body naturally lessens anger after about one minute.

When you understand this mechanism of the human body, you can apply it when your boss gets angry.

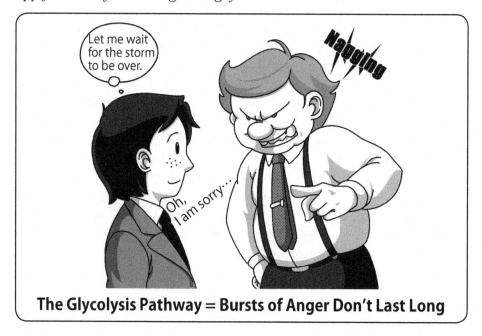

The Glycolysis Pathway = Bursts of Anger Don't Last Long

You should lay low and wait for the storm to be over, which should be in about one minute. Well, if your boss falls into hyperpnoea, then perhaps it lasts around two or three minutes.

Remember that bursts of anger lasts for about three minutes at the longest. You don't need to be twisted around your boss's fingers or further fuel new bursts of anger by talking back. Leave an angry person alone for 30 minutes and they will lose the energy to stay angry.

On the other hand, if we follow this logic and you want to scold someone with a huge display of anger, then you should first hold your breath until you turn blue and release your anger at once. If needed, then be furious at an appropriate time.

However, keep in mind that repetition of these fiery bursts brings hypoxia and hypothermia frequently. These conditions are not good for your body.

The world of hypoxia and hypothermia is also the world of cell divisions, which can encourage canceration of cells when the human body is exposed to high levels of stress.

In sports as well, if you only do sessions of intense training in the anaerobic environment, then your body falls into the energy production via glycolysis pathway and triggers hypoxia and hypothermia.

We humans are living beings who are able to survive longer when we implement aerobic exercises in our daily life. It allows us to use the mitochondrial pathway for energy production and utilize oxygen for growth.

If you want to achieve longevity, don't rely on instantaneous force too much. Place your foundation of daily life in the aerobic world, relying on energy production through the slower mitochondrial pathway. For this, it is also very important to learn to control your anger as well.

Living in a lifestyle where you snap at people easily is harmful for your interpersonal relationships. It is also harmful to cells in your own body.

Whenever we realize that we pushed ourselves too hard over our limit, we all should make efforts to leave the world of hypoxia and hypothermia and to regain the balance in our lives.

Here lies wisdom from the past: wisdom of deep breathing and keeping our body warm. This will create an environment where the mitochondrial pathway can be advantageous.

Importance of Cooling the Body for Men

Now, you probably understand the importance of escaping from a lifestyle which produces hypoxia and hypothermia. At the same time, please do not misunderstand and assume that the world of hypoxia and hypothermia is absolutely unnecessary to our life. Allow me to repeat myself: humans are equipped with two energy pathways, the glycolysis pathway and the mitochondrial pathway. It is not about which of them is better, but both of them are necessary in our lives. If we label the glycolysis pathway as evil and the bad one, then we will soon be unable to even get angry once in a while.

In my opinion, modern day individuals forget to get angry, to show emotions. If you encounter something unreasonable and unfair, you should get furious about it. That is the time when you use your instantaneous force produced by the glycolysis pathway wisely.

Otherwise, injustice in the society will not be corrected and all will be ignored and forgotten as if it has never happened. For example, if I lose my enthusiasm with age, then I will not be able to criticize modern medicine which has a lot of issues.

Modern medicine has labeled diseases as evil, and has advanced (or perhaps retrogressed) by seeking the removal of diseases. We cannot solve all diseases by just removing the bad parts. Also, stress is not evil. If you fear the state of hypoxia and hypothermia, that is also an overreaction.

As I mentioned a little bit in the previous chapter, for men, hypothermia is a necessary condition for cell division of sperm. In Japan, men participate while shirtless in many fertility-themed festivities, which have been in practice for hundreds and thousands of years.

Recently, a poster featuring a shirtless Japanese man with thick hair on his chest became popular in Japan. It was a poster about So-Min-Sai, a festival in the Iwate Prefecture. In the old days, they did not even cover their bottoms with fundoshi, a Japanese loincloth. It was not deliberately done to make these festivals unique, but by doing so, they were training the glycolysis pathways of men.

In Touka-Machi City in the Niigata Prefecture in Japan, people traditionally practiced "Muko Nage" in which people throw a groom into the snow from the main hall of a temple. From a medical point of view, it can encourage cell division of sperm; it might have carried the meaning of sending a warm farewell gift to a groom who will be having children soon.

In southern Japan where the climate is mild, people widely hold winter swimming events. Also, swimming in the winter is widely practiced around the world.

In Scandinavian countries, winter swimming is closely connected with their sauna traditions. People jump into a hole in a frozen lake and swim after sitting in a sauna that was built nearby. In Finland, there is an Avantouinti (ice-hole swimming) Society that maintains swimming holes for people who practice ice swimming in the winter.

Also, in Russia, people swim in the cold water of a frozen lake. Russians swim in cold water as a ritual of the Orthodox Church for the feast of the Baptism of Our Lord and for sports.

In Canada and in the U.S., members of the "polar bear club" go bathing outdoors or swimming in winter. The oldest ice swimming club in the U.S. is the Coney Island Polar Bear Club located in New York. They hold an annual 'polar plunge' on New Year's Day as well as regular sessions of winter swimming every Sunday from November to April.

People around the world had insights of making the glycolysis pathway advantageous. Our ancestors made full use of glycolysis pathways when they needed it and left strong descendants behind.

Also, the Nagano Prefecture which is located in a cold climate is always ranked among the top in average life expectancy. One of the countries ranked higher than Japanese men's life expectancy is Iceland, which is literally the Country of Ice.

Other countries that ranked higher than Japanese men are Switzerland, which have cold climates in high altitude and San Marino, a small country located in the mountain of Italy.

In addition, the cooling of testicles to increase men's sexual ability has been practiced since the old days.

However, people living in the modern day tend to be too serious and work too hard every day. People fall into chronic hypoxia and hypothermia, and have low level of health conditions. People weakened their ability to use the glycolysis pathway by living like the way many people live now, and consequently, people cannot utilize the glycolysis pathway even when they needed.

To summarize, the cause of cancer is also a lifestyle that cannot effectively use the glycolysis pathway.

Getting cancer when you become old is a result of an unbalance in your body, piling up to forming a cancer as you age.

By pleading to your doctor "Please treat the cancer," and exterminate cancer cells by having surgery or using chemotherapy do not change this unbalance in your body.

As people in the old days, it is more effective and important for you to reduce chances of cancer cell survivals by taking long warm baths or exercising to warm up your body to reduce stress that your body is experiencing.

In other words, yes, we should live the lifestyle while dominantly utilizing the energy produced via the mitochondrial pathway.

In the next chapter, let's think further about how to face stress. Stress can work both positively and negatively to our bodies.

From Abo Laboratory 2:
We Go Back and Forth Between "Two Ways of Living"

Please remember that there are two energy pathways within the 60 trillion cells that are within our bodies: the glycolysis pathway and the mitochondrial pathway.

When cancer proliferates, the glycolysis pathway becomes prominent. However, it is not correct to say that the glycolysis pathway is evil and bad for our bodies. Our bodies maintain daily activities by each pathway fulfilling its own role; the glycolysis pathway that is activated in the anaerobic environment and the mitochondrial pathway that is activated in the aerobic environment.

The mitochondrial pathway produces much larger amounts of energy, but individuals living in modern society are not making full use of the mitochondrial pathway. Many live an unbalanced, stressful lifestyle, which heavily relies on the glycolysis pathway (instantaneous force). Continuing to live such an unbalanced life can cause diseases by creating a continuous environment of hypoxia and hypothermia. It is important for all of us to realize this.

What is important is the balance in our lifestyle.

Chapter 3: True Role of Stress

Is Stress Evil?

In Chapter 1, I explained that cancer is not born because something is wrong within our bodies, but it is a normal adaptive response against the state of hypoxia and hypothermia.

Conditions of hypothermia and hypoxia, which may cause canceration of human cells, are the state where people are over-stressed. If it is hard for you to grasp how it feels to be in the over-stressed emotional state, then imagine how you would feel if you are completely lost in a jungle, alone.

In that state, there are many 'beasts' hiding in shadows, such as pressures from jobs and stressful interpersonal relationships with the people you work with.

To deal with these 'beasts', our bodies induce the state of hypothermia and hypoxia. By having the state of hypothermia and hypoxia, our bodies can respond to the emergency that is occurring with instantaneous force. In responding to such emergencies, it may also cause the canceration.

Many people may not realize such an adaptive response in our bodies, especially when they consider that "having cancer is a bad thing". It is also important to note that the over-stress may affect the Autonomic Nervous System (ANS). If you have read my previous books, you know that the ANS is consisted of two nervous systems: the Sympathetic Nervous System (SNS) which becomes dominant when our bodies are active and the Parasympathetic Nervous System (PNS) which becomes dominant when our bodies are relaxed and at rest.

When our bodies are exposed to stress, the SNS is at work. When we get irritated or let ourselves turn purple with rage, the SNS sends a command to release neurotransmitters (adrenalin, noradrenalin and dopamine) which can result in a faster heart rate, higher blood pressure and higher blood glucose level.

Neurotransmitters play major roles in the communication between nerves and other parts of the human body. The nervous system is not exactly like a power line, but a collective of scattered nerve cells. Neurotransmitters are chemical messengers which carry signals between the synapses, a tiny gap between one neuron to another. The following is a flowchart of how the SNS affects the hormones in our bodies:

Stress

↓

The Sympathetic Nervous System Becomes Dominant

↓

Neurotransmitters such as Adrenalin and Noradrenalin are Secreted

↓

Blood Vessels Contract, resulting in the Obstruction of Blood Flow

This is how our bodies fall into the state of hypothermia and hypoxia, which may lead to hyperglycemia and hypertension (high blood pressure). This process is not only supported by the SNS, but it is also supported by the hormonal system, especially since the hormones can affect the development of hyperglycemia.

In short, our bodies prepare to use the glycolysis pathway by making full use of the nervous system and the hormonal system.

In general, there is a common understanding that 'stress is not good'. However, having stress is a norm in our everyday lives. Our bodies respond to the stress, trying to adapt to the environment and trying to survive through it. As a result of such a response, we feel physical changes such as the loss of color in our faces and a faster heart rate caused by hypothermia and hypoxia.

These bodily changes are quite ordinary things in the human world.

However, continuing to have these conditions for a long period of time will cause diseases, because our bodies can only take so much stress. If we ignore the voices of our bodies and allow these conditions to continue further, then it may end in fatal illness.

When we look at the relationship between stress and diseases (which in the worst case scenario ends with the loss of life,) it reveals that there lies 'a mechanism to respond to the emergency in our bodies'. For example, wild animals will not survive an attack by its predators if their bodies use only the PNS and stay calm while they are being attacked. In reality, their SNS responds instantly, making the glycolysis pathway dominant to produce instantaneous force to respond to the emergency.

Stress is also necessary in some cases in our lives. So, it may not solve our health concerns when we focus on removing stress by considering that stress as an evil thing.

Also, both of the SNS and the PNS are important systems in our bodies. When the SNS is dominant, it does not always mean it is an unfavorable condition for the body, but it is a necessary body response to the given situation.

I believe it is important for us to look at each vital response as a part of the big picture, as the biological phenomenon. You may be surprised by finding a new meaning of the unfavorable condition when you look at it from the macro perspective.

Glycolysis Pathway's Response to an Emergency

To respond to an emergency in our bodies, the glycolysis pathway starts to operate at full capacity. As a result, the body falls into the state of hypothermia and hypoxia. This is an entire map of stress leading to hypothermia and hypoxia. To understand fully about how the glycolysis pathway works, I would like to add some more explanations about this pathway.

In Chinese characters, the glycolysis pathway is written as a "break down of carbohydrates (glucose)". It literally is a pathway which produces energy from nutrients. The main nutrient used to produce energy is carbohydrates. It is carried to the inside of cells via blood and then broken down to a substance called pyruvate near the cellar membrane.

Both glucose and pyruvate are in the sugar family, but glucose is a hexose whereas pyruvate is a triose. Energy is produced when a hexose is broken down into a triose.

It is a simple process of the carbon linkage separating. This process produces energy a hundred times faster than the complex process of the mitochondrial pathway. As I mentioned in the earlier chapter, the glycolysis pathway produces 2 molecular of energy in comparison to 36 molecular energy produced by the mitochondrial pathway. Even though the amounts of energy produced in the glycolysis pathway is 1/18 of the energy produced in mitochondrial pathway, the glycolysis pathway has an ability to produce energy quickly. This enables the glycolysis pathway to fuel the instantaneous power needed to respond to an emergency.

At the same time, this process produces lactic acid, a substance which makes us fatigued, while the pyruvate is being produced. Because of this, our energy does not last when we only rely on the glycolysis pathway for energy production.

It happens when we run at our full speed – we get tired very quickly. You can also visualize how lions are after they catch their prey.

Lactic acid is carried to the liver via blood. In the liver, glucose is re-produced. This glucose will be converted into energy by the mito-chondria within the muscles and liver. We inhale oxygen deeply and re-peatedly after racing at our top speed. This is because the mitochondrial pathway in our body needs lots of oxygen to convert lactic acid back to glucose. However, when we overwork the mitochondria in the liver, the liver itself can be burdened and weakened.

Also, blood becomes very viscous (sticky) when our bodies are un-der hypothermia and hypoxia. This is caused by the erythrocytes (red blood cells) combining with one another. It slows down blood flow – our bodies 'prepare for battle' when responding to an emergency in case blood will be shed. I will explain about this in detail in the later chapter.

In other words, the characteristics and textures of blood change in accordance with physical situations. This is an adaptive response. Our bodies are responding to the emergency.

As I mentioned earlier, energy produced by the glycolysis pathway can only last a short time. It may be only enough to respond to a low level stress.

Every time I discover how our bodies respond in accordance with different situations, I am moved by the wisdoms that dwell upon life. We need to first listen and understand the wisdoms within our human bod-ies to learn how to respond to diseases. Once we understand them, you will discover a new way of reacting and responding to diseases.

The glycolysis pathway may seem to be an ineffective energy path-way, but it plays an important role in responding to an emergency our bodies encounter.

Hyperglycemia is Also Caused by Stress

When we think that way, it may shed a new light in looking at the meaning of diabetes caused by hyperglycemia.

The causes of diabetes are commonly understood as high-calorie and high-fat diets as well as the lack of exercise. It is also understood that it has a strong correlation with obesity. This common understand-ing alludes to inconsistent lifestyles which prevent the body from func-tioning normally.-This chain of thoughts however, does not lead us to the core essence of an adaptive response.

When we focus on looking at the symptoms only, it may seem that the body failed to function normally. Having hyperglycemia is the vital response to get the glycolysis pathway to activate.

As I mentioned earlier when I explained about cancer, if we consider the glycolysis pathway's anaerobic exercise as a bad thing which causes cancers, then we may get lost in the path of finding the significance of having two different energy pathways in our bodies.

Both pathways are necessary for our bodies. These pathways have co-existed over 2 billion years since life started as prokaryotes. Both pathways have been utilized by living organisms since the beginning of their history. It is obvious that we need to be attentive about the 'method of utilizing' both pathways effectively, rather than thinking about which one is better than the other.

Daily diets and lack of exercise may also be triggers for hyperglycemia, but we lose the very core of the issue concerning stress when we only focus on diets and lack of exercise.

It may be obvious to you by now that **in the foundation of finding the causes of diabetes, we should take a look at "our bodies' adaptive responses to stress".**

In our bodies, when the SNS reacts to stress, adrenal glands secretes adrenalin and nerve endings releases noradrenalin. As a result, glucose in our bodies is carried into the blood stream, raising glucose levels.

At the same time, our bodies create a 'battle ready' environment with adrenaline rushing through our bodies, where the heart rate become faster and blood pressure increases. When stress increases, it increases the heart rate and our bodies respond to the stress by secreting hormones which increase the glucose level. As you can see, stress is a key component in this mechanism.

Modern medicine offers diabetic patients with dietary therapy and exercise therapy, but these have not been sufficiently effective so far.

In both therapies, people need to follow strict rules which create stress by continuing such therapies. Ironically, diligently following the rules by exercising and limiting what to eat may cause an increase in the glucose level.

Why is There a Low Rate of Obesity among Japanese?

Because of these reasons, it is in my opinion that dietary therapy, which is considered the most effective therapy for diabetic patients, is the 'second most important' treatment available for diabetes. I agree that it is a necessary therapy, but it is more important to deal with stress than the diet to improve the condition of hyperglycemia.

For example, when we eat sweets, the glucose level will rise but it does not mean that everyone who loves sweets have diabetes. Some people who have diabetes do not eat that many sweets either.

It is similar to people who can eat a lot but do not always have obesity.

In general, people who have obesity have a relaxed body type, whose PNS is dominant.

There are more Americans who fit in this body type than Japanese. I agree that in the case of obesity, it is necessary to have certain levels of control in what we eat.

However, it is important to note that many people who are serious and diligent workers can still gain weight. I believe that many become diabetic because the stress triggers the SNS which causes tension and results in hyperglycemia. **When conditions of hyperglycemia continue, then it can cause diabetes.**

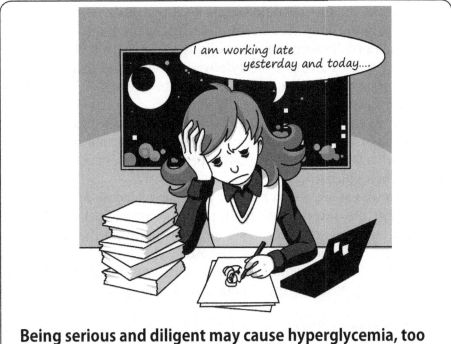

Being serious and diligent may cause hyperglycemia, too

To prove this, some Japanese are little heavy but they are not as large as some Americans with obesity.

Some people who feel a little heavy can be the types who have been relieving stress by eating. For them, the best way to face the issue is to re-examine what is causing their stress, stop overworking and having lack of sleep.

Please note that it may not mean that the same treatment options work for all patients just because all the patients have the same condition of diabetes. The same thing can also be said about the effectiveness of exercise therapy.

First, it is very important to understand the reasons why the glucose level increases. Let's go back to the relationship among the ANS, the hormones and glucose that I mentioned earlier.

It is the ANS as well as hormones that are maintaining the balance of the glucose concentration rate (glucose level). Adrenaline which increases the glucose level is secreted by the command of the SNS. In contrast, insulin which decreases the glucose level is secreted by the command of the PNS.

When we are tired by overworking or have extreme stress, the SNS become tense. In this condition, even feeling a little irritation over a small thing in the daily life can increase the glucose level.

In addition, the secretion of insulin is being controlled by the PNS. When people keep living a lifestyle where the SNS is dominant, then secretion of insulin is decreased - it may not be effective in reducing the high glucose level.

Many modern people lead very irregular lifestyles; often times the day and night is reversed. This can cause hypothermia and hypoxia. People with a low glucose level body type may try to get some sweets to increase their glucose level.

When we eat sweets on an empty stomach, glucose levels increase rapidly after digestion of sweets. In this case, people get energy for a while but our body also secretes a lot of insulin from the pancreas to respond to a rapid increase in the glucose level.

As a result, after a while the glucose level will start decreasing rapidly and people lose energy. Repetitions of this cycle will burden the body.

Glucose does not keep rising. It increases and decreases depending on different situations. Human bodies follow such laws of nature.

Modern medicine often focuses on the disadvantage of having hyperglycemia, and often suggests the importance of lowering the glucose level. They may only be looking at one side of a coin. In reality, the problem may be that the irregular glucose level is created by the inconsistent works of the ANS due to a stressful lifestyle.

There are so many more interesting facts about the relationship between eating and energy productions in the cells that I need to explain it in detail. I will explain about this relationship later in Chapter 8.

Relationship between Stress and White Blood Cells

To re-examine the relationship between stress and diseases, I would first like to explain about the relationship between the ANS and the immune system. The immune system defends our bodies from attacks by viruses, bacteria or cancer cells. One of the major components of the blood is White Blood Cells (WBC) which has an important role in maintaining the immune system.

Because of its role, WBC are also called defensive cells. There are many different kinds of defensive cells and all these cells work together to protect our bodies. Major players are granulocytes and lymphocytes.

Granulocyte is known to basically process the larger sized foreign substances, such as bacteria and dead cells.

Granulocyte makes up approximately 60% of the WBC which exists within the blood. Lymphocyte takes care of smaller sized foreign substances, such as viruses and cancer cells. Lymphocyte makes up 35% of the WBC.

In addition to granulocyte and lymphocyte, 5% of the WBC is being occupied by macrophages which eat bacteria and waste. Macrophages have the role of commander, controlling over the entire WBC.

We can consider that the ancestor of the macrophage branched out and differentiated into defensive cells.

I will explain now on how the WBC defensive cells work by giving you the prospect of having the flu as an example.

First, when the flu virus enters into our bodies, macrophages mobilize themselves to take action against the virus, eating the cells infected by the flu virus. However, that is not enough to protect the cell from the flu virus, so the macrophages then command the lymphocyte to produce antibodies which can catch the virus. This antibody will be launched from the B cell, one of the lymphocytes. The antibody will condense and catch the virus which is a pathogen (antigen). The virus will be consumed by the macrophages and granulocyte, and the foreign substance will be expelled.

Let's reflect this on the physiology of our bodies. We feel tired and have a fever, then that is a sign of lymphocytes working actively.

By increasing the body temperatures, our bodies activate lymphocytes to fight against the foreign substance.On the other hand, when watery nasal mucus becomes sticky, we would feel the yellowish purulent phlegm. That is a sign of the granulocyte cleaning up the pathogen and so on. Sticky purulent phlegm is actually the corpse of the granulocyte which fought with the pathogen.

My research revealed that these granulocytes and lymphocytes are controlled by the ANS. I also discovered the following rules (I call this finding the "Fukuda Abo Theory" as it was a collaborative research with Dr. Minoru Fukuda):

When the Sympathetic Nervous System is dominant
↓
Increased secretion of Adrenalin
↓
Increase the numbers Granulocyte

When the Parasympathetic Nervous System is dominant
↓
Increased secretion of Acetylcholine
↓
Lymphocyte is activated

In short, when our bodies are exposed to stress, the SNS becomes dominant which will increase the numbers of granulocyte. During the day when the SNS is dominant, there are more chances where our bodies sustain injuries and contract bacteria from wounds. Granulocyte is capable of catching and eating the larger sized foreign substances such as bacteria immediately.

On the other hand, during the evening and when we eat, smaller sized foreign substances such as viruses tend to enter our bodies. During these times, PNS becomes dominant. Deteriorated cells due to a whole day of activities and cancer cells tend to appear when we rest at night, too. Lymphocyte has a role promoting metabolism and attacking viruses effectively by producing antibodies.

Many Diseases are Responses to Stress

When our bodies are preparing for battle, defensive cells within the blood increase the numbers of granulocytes. By doing so, our bodies are by its instinct, trying to prevent blood loss and wounds.

However, when granulocyte attacks, it also releases Reactive Oxygen Species (ROS) and so on. This means when granulocyte increases too much, then it can damage healthy tissue cells.

When our bodies continue to feel stress, we use energy predominantly from the glycolysis pathway. The state of hypothermia and hypoxia continues in this environment which lays out perfect conditions for the cancer cells to proliferate. Increased ROS as a result of the increase in granulocyte can further encourage such proliferation of cancer cells.

By coordinating the works of the ANS, White Blood Cells (WBC) and energy production in the body cells, our bodies effectively deal with stress.

All these works are adaptive responses equipped inside of our bodies. Also, all of these are at work when our bodies are under the state of hypothermia and hypoxia. This is not a relaxing environment for our bodies. In addition, the glycolysis pathway is equal to instantaneous force, which means that it may overburden our bodies if these conditions continue.

In terms of the conditions of WBC, healthy numbers are when the granulocyte make up 50-65% and the lymphocyte consist of 35-41% of the WBC.

When I refer to a healthy condition, it also means that the SNS and the PNS are balanced. If you would like to live a relaxed life, then please keep in mind the importance of keeping the balance.

Please refer back to this book occasionally to reflect upon yourselves; if your current lifestyle is leaning towards either the SNS or the PNS, the glycolysis pathway or mitochondrial pathway.

The SNS is at work the whole time while our bodies are active. When we overuse it, it gets tense and it disturbs the balance of the ANS. It is my observation that people who live in the modern generation work too hard. Overworking results in the over-use of the glycolysis pathways. This will eventually lead to the over-working of the SNS.

When we were children, even if we run around and stayed active during the daytime using energy from the glycolysis pathway, we restored the balance of ANS after getting tired and resting in bed at night.

However, once we grow up and get a job, working hours increase and often times result in the reduction of sleeping hours. This means that the PNS does not have time to work, because our bodies are not resting. At a young age, people may still be able to handle this lifestyle. However, as we age and reach the 30's and 40's, it becomes harder and harder to live every day like this.

It becomes important then to make the PNS work and to move our body environment to the one where the mitochondrial pathways predominantly operate by taking sufficient rest.

If people decide not to do so, then, they will continue to spiral into the world of hypothermia and hypoxia. When this condition continues, it may lead to cancer. It could also lead to hyperglycemia and hypertension (high-blood pressure), which can cause various lifestyle related diseases, such as stroke and heart attacks.

I believe when our bodies are reacting to the stress, the process causes many diseases. Our bodies try very hard to respond to stress, and as a result it happens to cause diseases.

Reasons Why People Should Stop Working on the Frontline at their 40's

When people overwork all the time, sleeping hours will be reduced which can eventually create a lifestyle where days and nights are reversed. This can be an issue as well, because staying awake late at night induces SNS dominant condition. It will impose continuous stress and tension on our bodies, and will induce hypothermia and hypoxia.

For example, people who work at 24/7 operating convenient stores unintentionally induce a physical condition prone to cancer development. It creates the following conditions: the SNS becomes dominant leading to chronic hypothermia and hypoxia. In reality, I have seen some cases where young convenient store workers who worked the late night shift passed away from cancer.

Also, the same concept can be applied to factory workers who work night shifts. People who work night shifts all the time may want to consider changing the working hours to day shifts, so that the ANS is balanced. If the shifts cannot be changed, then try to be creative in finding alternative solutions. For examples, try to keep your body warm and enjoy your meal by eating slowly. By doing so, the PNS can become dominant.

As I mentioned earlier, when we are in our 20s, the glycolysis pathway is a main energy source. So, if people in their 20s work several night shifts in a row, their bodies can still overcome such situations. However, as people reach their 30's and 40's, the glycolysis pathways regress resulting in the inability to provide instantaneous force for dealing with continuous night shifts.

In addition, it is wise to leave the frontline of your work when you develop your professional career and become an experienced expert in the field. It is the best for your job performance and for your own health. For example, if you are a nurse who works at the hospital, then around the time when you are promoted to a head nurse, you should start re-examining your lifestyle. You should start relying on younger workers to do frontline jobs, such as directly taking care of patients or high caseloads by working in a demanding environment as in the Emergency Room. You should also stop working night shifts and start concentrating on taking care of your own body.

I will explain this in the next chapter in detail, **but after we reach 40's, it is better for our bodies to gradually shift from the lifestyle which relies on instantaneous force produced by the glycolysis pathways to the slower lifestyle which relies on the mitochondrial pathways.**

By changing the way of living your life, from the glycolysis pathway (instantaneous force) dominant body environment to the world of the mitochondrial pathway (endurance) dominant body environment, you can manage your stress better and have an opportunity to reflect upon yourself. Of course, by moving to the mitochondrial pathway dominant body environment, you will build foundations for "the way of life without cancer". For people who have a sense of strong responsibility and are hard-working in nature, when they are promoted in the management positions, they may keep working with their subordinates in the front-line which is considered a novel virtue. However, when we compare such virtues with the laws of life, then it is not a suggestible thing to do.

I would also call the laws of life as the voices of our bodies. If we ignore the laws of life by not being able to entrust frontline work to subordinates and keep working hard, then it leads us in ignoring our bodies' voices. If we keep ignoring the voices, then it will lead to hypothermia and hypoxia. Also, if the conditions of hyperglycemia continue, eventually body cells will lose its ability to function. These conditions will encourage the development of lifestyle diseases such as cancer.

Of course, these issues cannot be solved only by the efforts of individuals. It also has a lot to do with how society as a whole faces these issues. For example, if you are the owner of the company, it is very important for you to offer an effective working environment where each individual worker can flourish with their abilities and skills. If not, then the health of workers can be compromised. When this happens, the company as a whole loses its morale and productivity. Also, the increase of cancer patients will not ever change.

As I mentioned, I also agree that it is important to be mindful about having healthy diets and exercising regularly. However, these things are second in priority.

The fundamental reasons why we get diseases are hidden deep inside of ourselves. It is hidden inside of our way of thinking and the personal values we hold. You may feel that this is difficult to grasp and change if necessary, but the most important thing may be to change your mindset.

Living organisms have continued to survive by adapting to better ways to survive in given situations. Through a millions of years of struggles, we gained two energy pathways, the glycolysis pathway and the mitochondrial pathway.

By understanding characteristics and functions of two different kinds of pathways, and by learning its relationship between the ANS and stress, you will be able to discover how to gain a healthy lifestyle for yourself.

Not Too Diligent, Not Too Lazy

In previous chapters, we took a look at how our bodies can lose its balance by being exposed to stress. I also emphasized on the importance of having balance in your life in previous chapters. Balance is important in human bodies. I will explain this further, but avoiding even a tiny level of stress may not be good for our bodies. In other words, by entirely avoiding stress, this can also lead to getting diseases.

In short, when our bodies are over exposed to stress, then the SNS is burdened. When our bodies do not have exposure to even a small level of stress, then the PNS is burdened.

Overworking will lead to the continuous conditions of hypothermia and hypoxia. But when our bodies keep avoiding stress, metabolism can be suppressed, and this condition can also lead to having hypothermia.

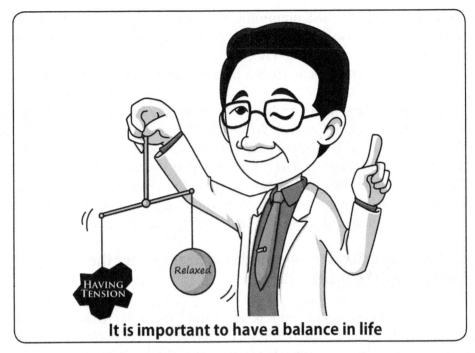

It is important to have a balance in life

In this condition, the lymphocyte might lose its activities which will lead to a loss of immunization strength.

For people who are always tense and excited, then it is important to relax and escape from the glycolysis pathways dominant conditions. However, for people who stay in all the time and live a slow, relaxed life every day, then it is important to get some butterflies in the stomach once in a while to get some tension back in their lives.

People who look very calm and seem to have a very relaxed, slow life without stress can have cancer, too. In this case, cause of cancer can be unbalanced lifestyle while heavily relying on the PNS. Such an unbalanced condition can lead them to a state of hypothermia and hypoxia.

Also, when people live a slow life without any stress, they lose their abilities and skills to manage things in their daily life. Consequently, trying to live a normal life can become stressful for them.

Breast cancer among women is increasing in recent years – not all the patients of breast cancer are overworking women who have led stressful lives. Some women have a very calm, relaxed life – these women also can have conditions for the development of cancer, as their metabolisms may have been lower due to their slower lifestyles.

In modern society, **about 70% of people who have some types of diseases are probably overworked, over-stressed individuals whose** body conditions are SNS dominant. The remaining 30% are opposite of this type, who do not have any stress at all, but their body conditions are predominantly the PNS.

I want to make it clear - it is a balance we need to keep in mind to attain healthy lifestyle.

Human beings maintain health by going back and forth between tense moments and relaxation. When this fine balance is compromised, then diseases may start appearing. When you understand this concept, then you will see how to wisely co-exist with stress. "Not too Diligent, Not Too Lazy"- finding and acquiring ways to maintain such a balance is a theme for leading a good life. When you find such balance, you can avoid having a major disease and enjoy aging year after year.

Diseases Give Good Opportunities to Learn About the Imbalance in Your Lifestyle

Now, let's change the point of view and look at the body parts that get cancer. Each patient has cancer in different parts of body. It is related to which parts of the body that was under the hypothermia and hypoxia. For example, people who get intense stomach pains when they get stressed probably have their stomach suffering from hypothermia and hypoxia. When this condition persists, then cells in the stomach starts proliferating rapidly which may cause stomach cancer.

As in the same concept, when you have so many concerns about your life and you feel out of breath all the time, then it may lead to lung cancer. If a person is very talkative, then that individual may be prone to get laryngeal cancer.

Of course, as I mentioned earlier, if a person leads a slow, over-relaxed life, then lower metabolism leads to obstruction of blood flow and can get cancers such as prostate cancer.

In general, the athletes who overuse the glycolysis pathway by intense trainings can have a tendency for prostate cancer. However, the lack of exercise can also lead the body to have the condition where PNS is dominant, which can also cause prostate cancer. Company executives who sit on executive chairs in comfortable executive suite offices tend to get prostate cancer, and this is probably caused by the over burdening of the PNS.

For these executives, I recommend them to deal with obesity by improving their metabolism. By having a lighter body, they will be able to gain a balanced body to use SNS effectively.

People who worry too much may induce hypoxia and hypothermia due to their mental stress. This may cause brain cancer.

When women with large breasts have breast cancer, the cause of cancer can be explained that the prominent breasts have cooled temperatures which promoted proliferation.

When we jog or jump ropes and move our bodies up and down, then the bone marrow is stimulated which can potentially lead to having myeloma or osteosarcoma. Surprisingly, standing and jumping can impose stress on human bodies.

Also, speaking of burdening the bone, myelogenous leukemia can happen to people who carry heavy things and occur when your work require long hours of standing.

In the past, a man in his 50's called me for consultation because he had myelogenous leukemia. When I listened to his situation, I learned that he had his own business which required him to stand all the time. Also, a Kabuki actor, Danjuro Ichikawa had the same cancer. A Kabuki actor wears heavy costumes that can weigh more than 20kg (≒44lb) for performing, so we can imagine how much of a burden the weight of the costumes placed on his body.

When these symptoms appear, we call them "site specificity" in the medical world. These symptoms appear because of an unbalanced lifestyle.

To sum up, **when we overuse particular parts of our bodies, stress will be cumulated in those parts. These overused parts will fall in to the state of hypothermia and hypoxia. When particular parts of your body get cancer, it is sign that you may need to change your lifestyle - how you live your life every day.**

It is not something mysterious that happens – there are reasons for the development of cancer.

Getting diseases can provide good opportunities for patients to re-examine the unique imbalance which exists in his or her life. It can give the person time to reflect on how he or she has lived so far and to obtain a clue to decide how he or she wants to live from now on.

I repeat – having imbalance in our lifestyle can happen to everyone. What is important is to know how the imbalance in our lives can show up in the diseases we get. Modify our lifestyles accordingly and by going through this process, we can teach ourselves a better way to live day by day. Having diseases give people opportunities to reflect on how they live and to know the self.

Usefulness of Stress

At the end of this chapter, I would like to add some more details on the ANS, as some misconceptions of the ANS exists.

Until now, I contrasted the roles of SNS and PNS to make it easier for you to understand. However, in reality, both of the systems work together as a team in our bodies.

As an example, please visualize when you play sports.

When we start moving our body, the cardio-respiratory function increases. It imposes stress onto our bodies and gradually, the SNS becomes predominant. As the length of the workout continues, it becomes tougher and tougher and at one point you may feel "I can't do it anymore".

However, after working out very hard, you rest and relax; the PNS gradually come to be dominant. As a result, you may gain the feeling of catharsis or a peaceful feeling.

In general, when we are calm, our pulse rate is 60 per minute. When athletes workout and take a break and relax, their pulse will slow down to 50 per minute, and sometimes even lower.

A lower pulse like this is often called an "athlete's heart". A condition of 50 pulse rate per minute is probably the place where these athletes can find peace. You might have noticed already, but this feeling of peace cannot be obtained if you don't work out very hard.

To sum up, **excitement and the feeling of peace, working hard and resting is both the back and front of a coin. When you understand these relationships, it becomes obvious to you that it is not about relaxing all the time which is the good way of living.** It may be an easy way of living, but in that way, people would not be able to appreciate the feeling of peace either.

To gain true peace of mind and happiness, it is also necessary to move our bodies and work out. By doing so, you may feel the joy of living your life.

When I say that the SNS and PNS are a team, what I mean is each system does not function independently. If we forget about this, then we will burden one of the nervous systems. Consequently, we will not be able to feel true peace of mind and happiness and we will lose the intricate balance between SNS and PNS. In addition, such imbalance may invite diseases and the feeling of illness signal us of that imbalance.

Of course, each person has his or her own capacity for exercising. Major League Baseball players such as Daisuke Matsuzaka, compared to a regular person have a different ability and capacity for exercising.

The stress level each person feels during exercise depends on each person's body type as well as one's physical ability. Understanding your own ability will help you determine balance when exercising. Such understanding will enhance the feeling of peace during the rest after exercising.

People who can easily finish 100 push-ups need to find the joy of life within that capacity. In contrast, there are people for whom doing 10 push-ups is difficult enough. It is important to know yourself.

Of course, this applies not only to sports but to many other scenes of our daily lives. To achieve one purpose in our lives will be accompanied by the exposure to stress, but feeling this stress is also a ticket to feeling joys and happiness at the end of the process.

Stress can induce hypothermia, hypoxia and hyperglycemia, which rely on the glycolysis pathways. It could pull people into having lifestyle related diseases and cancer. We gain happiness in life by effectively navigating through and balancing the stress in our daily lives.

Learning these things have made me say that the "normal range or normal value of hypertension may not exist" lately.

If a person has hypertension by living a normal way of life, then that reflects on the person's unique ability to do things briskly. He or she is probably a hardworking person. The person with this kind of personality should allocate a longer time to rest and sleep at night.

I am repeating myself again here, but I am not saying that life with stress is bad. In contrast, being lazy and just enjoying a life without stress cannot provide you with the feeling of fulfillment or happiness in your life, either.

In our bodies, a team of SNS and PNS, as well as a team of the glycolysis pathways and the mitochondrial pathways co-exist. It is important to use both teams in a balanced way. It is not so black and white in that we may say the glycolysis pathway is a hotbed for diseases so we should avoid using it; or we may say we should only depend on mitochondrial pathways or the PNS.

It is about finding your own true moderate ground – it is a difficult to find this, but by doing so, you will discover the meaning of joy and fulfillment in your life.

In the next chapter, I will answer the question of "what is a balanced life?" in detail by taking the lifetime of humans as an example.

From Abo Laboratory 3:
Re-Examine the Meaning of Stress

When living beings face an emergency, then our bodies respond to the stress by creating the state of hypothermia and hypoxia. Hyperglycemia can be also induced. These environments are burdensome for our bodies. Many doctors may focus on these conditions and try to treat these symptoms. When we take a step back and start to look at these conditions from a bigger picture, I believe it is apparent that these environments are our bodies' responses to emergencies that are happening to our bodies.

I have mentioned that when the state of hypothermia and hypoxia continues, then the glycolysis pathway becomes dominant in producing energy. The glycolysis pathway produces energy we can use instantly. Humans have survived difficult conditions by utilizing instantaneous force (the glycolysis pathway) since the beginning of its origin.

Please remind yourselves to have a second thought when you start thinking that there is something wrong with your body when you encounter these unfavorable body environments. It is our bodies' wisdom that creates these conditions.

However, it is also important to be mindful about not having our bodies continue to be exposed to these conditions. As these conditions continue, we naturally start having diseases. You may now realize that this also means switching to the mitochondrial pathway (endurance lifestyle) once in a while. It can be a good action to take, especially when you feel you have been under a lot of stress.

Chapter 4: What is a Balanced Lifestyle?

Wild Animals' Unbalanced Energy Pathways

As I explained so far, our bodies have two distinctive energy pathways. The glycolysis pathway has a simpler process for producing energy and the energy in this pathway is being produced instantly. The mitochondrial pathway has a complex process so it takes more time to produce the energy. I described the first one as instantaneous force and the latter one as endurance.

These two pathways co-exist within us, which mean that both pathways are necessary for functions within our bodies. The secret key to maintaining a healthy body and soul lies in how to use these pathways in a balanced way. Let me explain the reasons why it is important to use both pathways in a balanced way so that you will have a better understanding of the importance of doing so.

I will explain it by observing the activities of wild animals.

For instance, migratory fishes such as tuna, bonitos and mackerel cannot stay in one place. These fishes are called red fish and their endurance is highly developed, because their bodies consist of red muscles (slow muscles) which contain many mitochondria.

On the other hand, white fishes such as porgies and flounder drift on the waves or hide in the sand on the ocean floor. Only when they catch their prey, do they show their instantaneous force, capturing their target in one stroke. These fishes developed their white muscles (fast muscles) which contain few mitochondria, so they are good at moving instantly.

Similarly when we look at the energy production of birds, migratory birds such as wild ducks depend on the mitochondrial pathway to obtain endurance. Birds such as chickens that cannot even fly have energy productions which rely on the glycolysis pathway. In reality, wild ducks have a lot of red meat (red muscles) and chickens have a lot of white meat (white muscles). When we grill these birds and look at colors of their meat, the difference is obvious.

When we look at wild animals, carnivorous animals such as lions sleep all the time but catch their prey with a powerful instantaneous force. They are animals utilizing the white muscles with their energy production based on the glycolysis pathway. On the other hand, herbivorous animals such as cows and horses move slowly and have endurance. These animals probably developed red muscles and predominantly use the mitochondrial pathways.

The meat of cows and horses are red because they contain many mitochondria. When we compare their meat with color of chickens, the difference in color is pretty obvious.

When we look at the meat produce section at the super market, there is even a difference between Kobe (Japanese) beef, American beef and Australian beef in their color. Usually, American and Australian beef are redder than Kobe beef. Mitochondria increase in number when animals exercise. We can assume that American and Australian beef are redder in their color because these cows are pastured on the farm and get to exercise. American and Australian beef usually taste richer so they are good for steak when cooked.

Since Japanese cows do not exercise a lot, Kobe beef loses its color. The taste is not as rich, so Kobe beef are good when thinly sliced and used for dishes like shabu shabu. Kobe beef may be bland in taste when it is compared with American and Australian beef but their tenderness is superb.

Humans Are the Most Balanced Beings

Even when the animals belong to the same family, they can be one-sided in using one pathway for energy production, either predominantly using the glycolysis pathway or the mitochondrial pathway.

They do not completely rely their energy production on only one pathway, but by using one pathway more often, they adapt to the environment they live in to survive.

How about humans, then? Of course, some people are better at one thing than others, but humans can sprint 100 meters which require instantaneous force, and can also run a 40 kilometers marathon which requires endurance.

To better understand this, the following formula is ideal for maintaining the balance in our body environment:

Glycolysis Pathway : Mitochondrial Pathway = 1 : 1

As this formula shows, humans are the most harmonious beings among all the animals.

It may sound strange when I say that humans are the most harmonious (balanced) of creatures because we are the ones who destroy nature the most and thus damage many wild lives. But, our bodies have the ability to utilize both of the energy pathways. Most of us do not need to be taught to use these two energy pathways in harmonious and balanced ways, because it comes naturally to us.

To better understand this, I would like to look at a human life from when we are born.

When we are born, the glycolysis pathway independent to oxygen is mostly at work to encourage cell divisions. Interestingly, humans barely have mitochondria when we are born. When humans start pulmonary respiration, the numbers of mitochondria start to increase. When we reach about three years old, the measure of mitochondria in our bodies reach high numbers.

As we say "A three year old's soul lasts until the child becomes one hundred years old", human bodies repeat cell divisions until we reach three years old. Main organs such as the brain and heart are formed and intelligence level increase. The foundation of the person is formed around this time.

People still grow after reaching three years old, though not as rapidly as they did up to that point. When we turn fifteen years old, the growth of human beings more or less finishes. When mitochondria increase in number, the gene the mitochondria brought to human bodies which suppress cell divisions, start to work and suppress cell divisions in our bodies.

To be precise, sperm, skin, hair, bone marrow and intestinal epithelium continue in the division of cells, but the cell divisions stop for other parts of the human bodies, decreasing the use of the glycolysis pathway. As this change occurs, gradually, aerobic exercises utilizing the mitochondrial pathway become more predominant. The cells which repeat cell divisions have very few mitochondria.

When we understand the mechanism of human growth, we can easily understand the reasons why children are always energetic.

Young children utilize the glycolysis pathway's anaerobic exercises often, and they have plenty of instantaneous force to use. They would run around when they have a little chance, but even though they can jump and run, they are not good at running long distances.

Children may get bored easily, and they may play at full force though they get tired when it is time for them to clean up. When humans reach puberty, the mitochondrial pathway become more dominant, thus people start to calm down as well.

When mothers understand this, then they should not worry too much about the powerful energy that their kids have. Having instantaneous force is a natural thing for children due to the glycolysis pathway's dominance in fueling their energy. If mothers try to force their children to calm down, that may not work.

It is fine for mothers to accept that kids play loudly. By doing so may even allow mothers to decrease their irritation level and increase the feeling of love towards their children.

When kids calm down, that means that their energy productions change from utilizing the glycolysis pathway predominantly to mainly utilizing the mitochondrial pathway, indicating that young children have grown into adulthood.

Reasons Why the Lifestyle Changes in Accordance with Age

The energy production ratio between the glycolysis pathway and the mitochondrial pathway changes slowly. It varies from one person to another, but in general, during the ages between 20s and 50s, the energy production ratio between the glycolysis pathway and the mitochondrial pathway becomes 1:1, achieving harmonious balance between these two pathways. Our lives are the most productive during these 40 years, because we can utilize both the glycolysis pathway and the mitochondrial pathway in a balanced, harmonious way.

For example, in Japan, we have what we call "Wakage No Itari (youthful passion)", which describes how young people can lose their tempers easily or become passionate easily. People become composed and calm as we age and as a result, we can judge things better.

After reaching middle age, people tend to become more understanding of others and react to situations more calmly. Around this time, in our bodies, the mitochondria pathway become dominant. Movements of our bodies become slower, so people may lose the quick physical motions they had when they were younger.

Around the time when people reach their 60s, the human bodies start relying predominately on the mitochondrial pathway. At the end, there is death.

When I was younger, I remember I would lose my temper more easily. I remember kicking chairs around and would direct my anger toward my students. I calmed down around when I reach my 50s. I suppose my body started to increasingly rely on the mitochondrial pathway for energy productions then.

Around this time, I discovered that "The Autonomic Nervous System (ANS) controls the immune system". I applied my discoveries to my lifestyle as well. I reduced over-eating and increased my sleeping hours. I tried to use the Parasympathetic Nervous System (PNS) predominantly by changing my lifestyle. Due to these efforts, I feel that I calmed down a bit, but how I changed my mind to adapt to a new lifestyle itself came naturally, followed the laws of nature.

I am in my 60s now. When I continue to follow the natural ways of aging, my body will increasingly become dependent on the mitochondrial pathway for energy production. I would need to take in a lot of oxygen and would better lead a slower lifestyle. In this way, I would probably not get sick, but mature and age slowly.

In other words, if people at my age are still trying to live in a way they lived when they were younger, and continue to rely mostly upon the glycolysis pathway for energy production, it may create the continuous state of hypothermia and the hypoxia. These conditions may lead to various lifestyle related diseases such as cancer.

To live your life in such a way brings pain and suffering at the time when people should be enjoying their retirement. After working so hard for their entire life to reach the point, people should relax and have good time when they retire.

You may think pain and suffering comes with age naturally, but you certainly do not wish that is what awaits you when you retire. It is important to understand nature's providence, and shift our lifestyle from the glycolysis pathway dominant lifestyle to the mitochondrial pathway dominant lifestyle as we age.

An Ideal Formula for the Most Balanced and Harmonious Existence

=

1 : 1

Glycolysis Pathway: Mitochondrial Pathway

↓

Relationship between Energy Pathway and Age

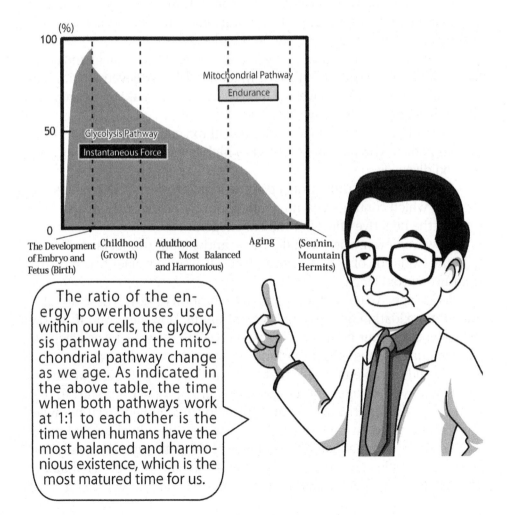

The ratio of the energy powerhouses used within our cells, the glycolysis pathway and the mitochondrial pathway change as we age. As indicated in the above table, the time when both pathways work at 1:1 to each other is the time when humans have the most balanced and harmonious existence, which is the most matured time for us.

Two Ways of Aging

Of course, we will eventually need to face death even if we do not get serious diseases. It is our destiny to face death after all.

The mitochondrial pathway which requires oxygen to produce energy can help us achieve longevity but at the same time, it can encourage aging by oxidation.

This is an inevitable process in all human lives. As humans, we start growing by cell divisions in the anaerobic environment. Then, we start to mature and age by shifting to rely on the mitochondrial pathway for energy production. Finally, we face death by aging further by oxidation.

I would like to go back to what I explained in Chapter 2, the story about how our human cells which originated from a bacterium equipped with aerobic mitochondrial pathway, started to live on a unicellular organism that was surviving solely on the glycolysis pathway.

Unification of anaerobic bacteria (our ancestral organism) and aerobic bacteria (ancestral organism of mitochondria) achieved our human evolution. However, we have not yet succeeded in making oxygen entirely harmless to human bodies.

I mentioned earlier about how radical oxygen are produced in the human bodies when we are exposed to high levels of stress, causing aging and diseases.

Our bodies naturally produce antioxidant enzymes, but by consuming food which contains vitamin C and E or phytochemical can also help remove the negative effects of radical oxygen.

However, even when we take these antioxidant products and try to fight the oxidation of the body, we will age as we grow older because that is nature's providence.

As we age, we get wrinkles and discoloration of skin. These are also related to oxidation and are the signs of aging. However, even if we try to look younger, our bodies will never go back to the way it was when we were at our 20s. It is also important to accept the fact that we age.

I would like to emphasize that there are two ways in how we age.

One way is the aging process where energy productions start to rely on the glycolysis pathway first and shifts to the mitochondrial pathway more and more as we get older. After a while, the mitochondrial pathway becomes dominant, and the balance of the pathways eventually collapse and people age consequently. This is the natural process of aging. You will lose the quickness and instant power you had when you were younger, and oxidation will continue slowly but surely and you will live out your natural life eventually.

The other way is the aging process where people use the glycolysis pathways all the time by leading stressful lives such as by overworking.

People age in this way live an unbalanced lifestyle even in the most balanced period when their bodies had the balanced and harmonious state where the glycolysis pathway and the mitochondrial pathway worked at the 1:1 ratio. People who lead this kind of lifestyle may easily fall into the continuous state of hypothermia and hypoxia, and can have the tendency to get various lifestyle related diseases such as cancer and diabetes.

Also, overworking the glycolysis pathway can burden the mitochondrial pathway as a consequence, because as I mentioned already, the mitochondrial pathway process the lactic acid created by the glycolysis pathway.

When you are at the age between 20s and 50s, during the time when humans have the most balanced and harmonious existence, take a good rest if you overworked or exposed your bodies to stress. By doing so, our bodies can maintain the balance between the glycolysis pathway and the mitochondrial pathway, as well as the balance between the SNS and the PNS.

If we are not mindful about keeping the balance, we age by exposing our bodies to stress.

In the past, there was a theory called "Aging by the Mitochondria Theory" which explained that the aging of the organisms are connected to the mitochondrial pathway. In fact, it is the overuse of the glycolysis pathway (anger, over-working, and being too diligent) that causes the aging. The mitochondrial pathway is just involved in the process.

These rules of life can provide us with starting points of thinking what is the best way to live our lives.

Why Do Kids and Elderly Persons Eat Differently?

When our bodies shift from using the glycolysis pathway for energy production to using the mitochondrial pathway, the change affects our daily diet as well.

For example, when we were kids, we get hungry quickly because we move around constantly while we are awake, using the energy produced primarily by the glycolysis pathway. Especially when kids are in their growth period, it is not enough to eat three meals a day. They would require eating snacks between meals as well. The energy produced in the glycolysis pathway is not efficient energy so kids need to eat more to fuel for their daily activities.

Even when adults think that kids are eating too much, the kids may not become obese or even have stomach aches after they eat.

Of course, kids can become obese when they do not play outside to release the energy they obtained from the glycolysis pathway. When kids read comic books at home or play video games all the time instead of running around outside, there will be leftover energy not being used and they can gain weight. As long as children play like they naturally do, we do not need to worry about them overeating. The energy converted from the food they eat will be consumed naturally.

As we grow out of childhood and reach our 20s and 30s, the mitochondrial pathway gradually becomes the primary source of energy, while decreasing the dependency on the glycolysis pathway for energy production. As this change happens, we do not need to eat so often, such as snacks. When we over-eat at this age period, unless we use the glycolysis pathway by exercising like sport athletes, we may still have leftover energy not being consumed which can eventually lead to obesity and cause various diseases.

When we reach the middle age, we eat foods even less as the mitochondrial pathway becomes more prominent in our bodies. We would not want to eat oily foods, and may start to prefer eating fish and beans instead.

At last, when we reach old age, we may lose the desire to eat and end up eating less and less. We may not need to eat snacks, not mentioning that we probably may not need to eat three meals a day. This situation is similar to the eating habits of the mountain hermits, as they are said to eat the mist in the air.

We hear every day about various opinions on what foods are good for us and there seem to be so many different ways to eat the right foods. When we look at the daily diet from the physiological view however, it is clear that the truth is that humans eat foods differently at a certain age.

We do not continue one way of eating for a lifetime – it changes. If we ignore that, then we will be forcing our bodies to accept an inappropriate way of eating. Ignoring the proper way of eating will not be good for our bodies regardless if we are eating nutritious foods or not.

For example, many people have been mentioning the importance of eating breakfast every morning. Eating breakfast is very important for young children, as children use the energy produced via the glycolysis pathway.

When we reach adulthood and become elderly, then it may be necessary to skip breakfast once in a while to prevent overeating. However, for kids, it is important for them to eat breakfast, to grow by making full use of the glycolysis pathway's works.

For kids, it is fine for them to eat until the parents feel they are bit over-eating. They should eat a big breakfast before going to school so that they can fuel their energy from food using the glycolysis pathway. This may also help the kids to get better grades since the glucose will reach their brain cells. The habit of eating has a connection to converting the nutrients to energy for daily activities within cells. It is important to understand the mechanism of how the conversion of the energy works within our bodies at different ages when we look at our eating habits.

It is a law of nature that kids and elderly persons eat differently as the energy production dependency shifts from the glycolysis pathway (when we were kids) to the mitochondrial pathway (when we are older). It is good to keep in mind that there may not be only one nutritional science that can apply to all people at different ages.

True Meanings of "Hara Hachi Bun Me – Eat Moderately"

Ekiken Kaibara (1630 - 1714), a Confucian scholar in Edo period, introduced Syoku Yo Jyo or Diet Regimen which taught a way of having a balanced diet for maintaining health. What is explained in Syoku Yo Jyo may be applicable after people pass their middle age.

Ekiken suggested "80% Diet" in his book called Yo Jyou Kun. 80% Diet means eating modestly until you feel 80% full. It is a fundamental way to depart from depending on the glycolysis pathway for energy production.

Basically, he preached that "when you get older, change your way of eating to the one suited to the mitochondrial pathway. Then, you will be able to achieve longevity in accordance with nature's providence."

Nanboku Mizuno (1757 - 1834), a physiognomy scholar in Edo period further developed Ekiken's Diet Regimen.

When he was young, he was a short-tempered person who enjoyed drinking sake, gambling and fighting. His lifestyle was a typical lifestyle where people overburden the glycolysis pathway.

One day, he was told by an old monk who practiced physiognomy, "Your face shows the sign of death. You will die within a year if you continue to live the way you live now." Then he made up his mind to change his lifestyle and only ate barley and soybeans for the entire year. As a result, the signs of death disappeared from his face and his mind calmed down. His luck said to be also increased after changing his lifestyle.

By changing his diet, he successfully escaped from the environment where he overused the glycolysis pathway, and shifted to using the energy produced via the mitochondrial pathway.

He left quotes such as "eating is life" and "eating can determine your destiny". It is true that eating habits can change how we live.

When we start depending on the mitochondrial pathway for energy production and have endurance, we become more relaxed, less temperamental and have the capacity to think deeper. When we live that way, our breath becomes deeper and longer, enabling us to take in a lot of oxygen. As the mitochondrial pathway becomes dominant, our bodies do not require so many intakes of nutrients. As a result, our bodies will feel great and we get sick less often.

When our bodies feel good, we feel happier which will bring good luck. You can see how eating habits can change one's life.

People who obtained the highest enlightenment of utilizing the mitochondrial pathway are the people we call Sen'nin, immortal hermits of the mountain.

Sen'nin, mountain hermits, are believed to eat the mist in the air. When people learn the way to maximize the use of the mitochondrial pathway, it really does not require much food. You may feel that it is unrealistic, especially when we look at this from a nutritional science point of view. It is actually not so mystical. I will further explain about this in detail in Chapter 8, but in short, I can sum it up in one statement: **The nutritional science's concept of "maintaining life by eating foods" is based on using the glycolysis pathway and is an unbalanced way of looking at the eating habit of humans.**

In reality, high monks used to decrease the amounts of foods they ate to obtain a clearer mind, and at the end they died from fasting. When we reach old age, we eat very little. The way for the high monks to die from fasting perhaps was natural and a fulfilling way to depart from life.

On the other hand, modern medicine keeps elderly patients who are bedridden alive by providing nutrition via intravenous drip (infusion) and tries to bring them back to utilizing their glycolysis pathways. Also, modern medicine will insert a tube into an elderly person's stomach who has gastrostoma. The person who has gastrostoma cannot eat on their own, so the doctors will send nutrients and water directly to the stomach by using the feeding tube.

Feeding tube treatment is probably done because modern medicine believes that sending nutrients to the human bodies is the way to maintain our lives. However, this method does not recognize that the bodies probably do not require the use of the glycolysis pathway any longer.

Usually, when people become bedridden and start eating less and less, it is a treasuring time for them to reflect upon their lives, being grateful for the lives they had while relying on the mitochondrial pathway for energy production. This is the natural way.

However, when patients are forced to live in a way in order to use energy from the glycolysis pathway again, and need to take painkillers, patients may fall into the spiral of being unhappy, feeling resentment or thinking ill of someone. Eventually that will lead to bewilderment which can end someone's life in an unhappy way.

When we understand that elderly people rely on the mitochondrial pathway for their energy production when reaching the end of their lives, it is easy to start realizing how silly it is to keep feeding nutrients and water to elderly patients.

Wild animals follow the flow of natural law without being taught to do so – they live and die naturally.

Is Terminal Care Necessary?

Since we are talking about eating now, I would like to introduce surprising works of the human bodies in processing nutrients.

When nutrients are absorbed by our bodies, the nutrients are carried to the cells via blood vessels and lymph fluid. When we eat too much, then the glucose that was not used will remain within the blood. One of the defensive cells, macrophages process these surplus nutrients left behind within the blood. The thinner people are, less macrophages will be in the blood.

This is because people who eat a lot require more macrophages to process the nutrients. When people do not usually eat a lot are forced to eat a big bowl of rice, they will feel difficulty. The lessened numbers of macrophages is the cause of this.

Even for a healthy person, being forced to eat a big bowl of rice can be painful. Imagine how painful it will be for a person who is at the end of their life and forced fed.

Some people may think that it is painful when we all die, but when we live in accordance with the law of nature, a peaceful death is possible for all of us.

In modern day society, many people are living in the lifestyle which depends on the glycolysis pathway to produce instantaneous force for them. Perhaps, because of that, we are caught up in a point of view of the glycolysis pathway.

However, when living beings die, the energy from the glycolysis pathway has already disappeared and they die quietly as plants die in nature. Animals also die this way in the wild. They die by shutting down the energy from the glycolysis pathway and keeping the last strings of life by using the energy from the mitochondrial pathway. By the time it comes to the end, we may stop inhaling the oxygen and quietly die.

Reasons why people living in the modern age cannot accept this natural way of dying is perhaps related to the value toward life and death which focuses on living only.

People may be fixated on living because they are afraid of the pain and suffering associated with death. But not all deaths accompany pain and suffering. Also, when we are in pain and suffering when we get diseases, that is not a wrong occurrence. Instead, our bodies are trying to adapt to an environment which we are exposed to.

By understanding this intricate balance of life, I hope you will transform your image of death. Living and death are the head and tail of a coin, and you do not need to be afraid of only one side of the coin.

I, myself, wish to spend the next ten and then twenty years by accepting the mitochondrial pathway's lifestyle and eating less food as the years go by, and eventually would like to accept my death in peace.

If you are taking care of elderly family members at home, you may want to think about the law of nature that I mentioned, and think about the necessity of terminal care. I understand that you want to do everything you can do for your family members. However, by providing too much terminal care, it may cause substantial suffering to the patients themselves.

You can finally discover the true meaning of death as the nature's providence when we understand the relationship between the glycolysis pathway and the mitochondrial pathway.

Overeating Can Weaken the Immune System

When we live naturally, our lifestyles shift from the glycolysis pathway dominant lifestyle to the mitochondrial pathway dominant lifestyle. In this process, you will naturally start to eat less and less as you age.

However, when people live in the glycolysis pathway dominant lifestyle during the period when their bodies require the harmonious balance between two pathways, the balance in their lives is lost and this may lead to the increase risk of obesity and lifestyle related diseases.

The reasons why fasting is believed to be good for the body is that it is effective in refining the balance by fixing the dependency to the glycolysis pathway.

Also, it will decrease the necessity of the macrophages to process the nutrients, thus the macrophages can focus on defending the body against foreign bacteria and virus. This is how our immune system is strengthened when we do not eat.

In reality, when we observe via microscope the macrophages which are summoned to take care of the leftover nutrients, they look so big and too heavy to move around. These macrophages are called foam cells and they will not be able to function as defensive cells.

Nutrients from foods are necessary for our bodies, but when we consume too much, it can decrease the immune system, causing us to get diseases. If you feel that you tend to overeat, it is a good idea to incorporate fasting to regain the balanced way of living your life.

Of course, even if fasting is good for our bodies, it requires limiting the food intake which we have been accustomed in having every day, so it may take a while to get used to the fasting.

I did a fasting experiment at my laboratory, and I realized my students and I could get irritated easily and become angry over small things after not eating three meals. Until the body gets used to it, the glycolysis pathway demands the intake of the nutrients, so you may find it difficult to control your feelings and heart.

Humans are made to feel satisfaction when we eat a feast. It is true that when the glycolysis pathway is the main source of energy production, irritation and anger weakens. Forcing yourself to continue fasting can be harmful to your body, and can cause severe hypoglycemia. If you continue fasting for a long time without having any proper guidance from an experienced person, in the worst case scenario, it can also lead to death.

Fasting is in a way of perfecting in advance the mitochondrial pathway dominant lifestyle which awaits you in the future. So, do not force yourself, but be conscious about getting used to the fasting gradually by training your own bodies to adjust. In a way, fasting can be said to be like training. Over-training can collapse the balance of the body so it is the same concept here for fasting as well.

Importance of an Appropriate Lifestyle for Your Age

You might have realized by now, but talking about how we live our lives at an old age and how our bodies prepare for a peaceful death overlap with the enlightenment that the religious world explains. So, at the end of this chapter, I would like to approach the subject of enlightenment from a scientific viewpoint.

What disciplinants of religions seek is, simply said, the peaceful life led by the mitochondrial pathway's lifestyle utilizing the aerobic exercises. Breathing exercise and modest eating habits allow them to emancipate from all kinds of desires that the glycolysis pathway's lifestyle offers.

It is true when we use energy mainly from the mitochondrial pathway, people calm down and lose their aggressions. Feelings like anger, sorrow, frustration and bewilderment belong to the world of hypothermia and hypoxia, so escaping from these feelings brings us to the path to peacefulness, which also will activate the mitochondrial pathway and lead us to longevity.

It has a significant meaning to approach a peaceful world toward the end of our long lives after experiencing so many things. For younger people, consciously leading a slower lifestyle will provide them with mitochondrial pathway dominant lifestyle. Younger generation also need to have a peacefulness in their daily lives once in a while.

However, to flip the coin to the backside, it means to lose worldliness and youthfulness. If you seek enlightenment when you are young during the time when you should be utilizing the glycolysis pathway, it may cause an energy imbalance and you may affect well being of your soul.

I am repeating this point again, **but what is important is to choose an appropriate lifestyle for your age.** The healthy balance of body and soul is connected to the balance between the glycolysis pathway and the mitochondrial pathway.

Please remember once again that when both pathways are at work in a balanced way, that is when body cells are at the most harmonious state.

A balanced, harmonious state means when the ratio of energy production by the glycolysis pathway and the mitochondrial pathway is 1:1 in our bodies. If we think of the glycolysis pathway as a bad pathway, then we will not be using half of the potential abilities in our bodies. When we become strict about choosing only one side, then we also fall from the laws of nature.

People will reach enlightenment when we age and naturally shift toward the mitochondrial pathway dominant lifestyle. Until then, what we can do is to live in our societies to play our daily roles, and be conscious about balancing the use of both pathways.

You should not avoid your desire for money, honor and sexual drives entirely.

When you are younger, remember what Dr. William Clark said. Dr. Clark made an impact in Japanese culture by establishing Hokkaido University in late 19th Century in Japan. After a brief stay in the island of Hokkaido, he said following parting words to his Japanese students: "Boys, be ambitious!" When you are young and feel drives and desires to live in human societies, then make good use of the energy produced by the glycolysis pathway, and be ambitious and be successful.

When you push yourselves too much, you may get sick. Getting sick itself is not a bad thing, but it is a way of life. While utilizing the instantaneous force to challenge many things in your life, make sure to rest and take a break sometimes by listening to your bodies and feelings. By doing so, when you get older, you will finally be able to appreciate the value of a mitochondrial pathway dominant lifestyle.

From Abo Laboratory 4:
Getting Sick is Another Result of Two Pathways Co-existing

So far, I explained in detail about two pathways, the glycolysis pathway and the mitochondrial pathway equipped within our cells.

Some of you might felt that "The mitochondrial pathway which can produce massive energy is superior to the glycolysis pathway". However, both pathways are necessary for our bodies as energy pathways. If you forget about this important point, your lifestyle may lose balance and you may not be able to fully utilize the abilities in your life.

I explained that the ideal formula for maintaining the most balanced life is when the ratio of the energy productions by glycolysis pathway and the mitochondrial pathway is 1: 1. However, when I mentioned 'balanced', I don't always mean to label this state as healthy. Remember, both of being healthy and being sick are necessary functions for our bodies.

When we can depart from the idea that "getting disease is a bad thing" and obtain the ability to accept the vital responses in our bodies as they are, then we will be able to clearly understand what true harmonious balance means.

Chapter 5: Uncommonly Known Differences between Men and Women

Reproduction Originates from the Union of Cells Occurring Two Billion Years Ago

I have explained so far that our bodies have two powerhouses. In this chapter, let's take a look at them in the context of sex.

Humans have two different sexes, male and female. A man and a woman produce offspring together and DNA information is inherited from one generation to the next in this way. Everyone probably knows about this, but many do not know how the distinction between male and female came about.

The key to uncovering this is also held by the two powerhouses, the glycolysis pathway and the mitochondrial pathway.

Protocell (prokaryote), which could only proliferate by cell divisions in the beginning, achieved dramatic evolution by taking in the aerobic bacteria. The aerobic bacteria's ability to convert the oxygen into energy was very helpful to them because the environment with oxygen was a harmful environment to the protocell.

As you now know, these aerobic bacteria became mitochondria later on. One human cell can carry from hundreds to thousands of mitochondria.

Life obtained a ticket to remarkable evolution, reaching the level of higher organisms like humans by obtaining mitochondria, which could process oxygen that many other organisms could not process.

An important point to remember here is when life obtained the ability to grow by utilizing oxygen, it also embraced the process of aging and death at the same time.

Protocell uses a simple energy production system to survive, and does not go through the process of growth or evolution even though they may go through some changes. Life (eukaryote) entered into the process of growth and aging when it obtained the mitochondria and its ability to produce massive energy.

You may think that growth and aging as opposite concepts, but by obtaining the energy from oxygen, humans started to go through the process of growth and oxidation, which naturally results in aging.

Down the line of the human growth spectrum is aging, and at the end of it is death. This became the destiny of the organism which achieved evolution.

Higher organisms could not leave descendants by just growing and aging. So reproduction, the process of producing offspring by the union of two organisms was born to serve that purpose.

Reproduction can take different forms and to be precise, the cell divisions in the glycolysis pathway are also counted as reproduction (asexual reproduction). However, what I am going to talk about now is about sexual reproduction which is achieved by the unification of male and female, the sperm and ovum.

Both the sperm and ovum are in charge of reproduction. They are parts of the cell that have roles of bridging DNA information from one generation to the next.

A very interesting fact about these reproductive parts is that each sperm and ovum only leaves half of their chromosomes.

Animals unite sperm and ovum by copulation, and half of the chromosomes from the sperm and the ovum are united in the ratio of 1:1. It means that the animals inherit DNA information from both the male and female.

Plants unify by the stamen, the male reproductive part touching the pistil, the female reproductive part. Plants too, inherit the DNA information from both the male and female reproductive parts equally.

Reproduction of organisms started from the unification of two distinctive cells, and till this day organisms leave descendants to the next generation in this way.

Some of you might have realized now that in fact, **reproduction originated from the union of cells (anaerobic bacteria with the glycolysis pathway and the aerobic bacteria with the mitochondrial pathway) which occurred 2 billion years ago. To solve the mysteries of the mating between women and men, we needed to go back to that time.**

Mitochondria is a Feminine Organelle

When we understand the mechanism of organisms, we can also find an answer to what it means to be a man or a woman.

Let's take a look at the inside of the nucleus of a human cell. The nucleus of a human cell has 23 pairs of chromosomes and each carries DNA which contains genetic information. However, there is an exception.

Mitochondria in the cell carry its own DNA, too.

The DNA in mitochondria is considered as evidence of the mitochondria being an external organism (aerobic bacteria) once in the past. Even though the mitochondria have its own DNA, it does not mean that the mitochondria can function independently away from the human body.

Mitochondria, an organelle, shifted most of its DNA into the nucleus to suppress unnecessary cell divisions.

Mitochondria produce energy from hydrogen in return for borrowing the DNA information from the nucleus. This is how mitochondria and host cells (the human cell) have been co-existing.

The interesting thing is that only the maternal side of mitochondria's DNA information is transmitted to the next generation. The fertilized ovum inherits DNA information only from the ovum which contains tremendous numbers of mitochondria.

So, when we go back in history, the DNA of the mitochondria leads to one ancestor, a woman.

Going back to about 1.5 hundred thousand years ago, we can find the ancestor of all mankind, an African woman who was given a name, Mitochondria Eve.

We discovered that by trying to find the origin of mitochondria. Humans originated in Africa and from there, we had spread around the globe.

The mitochondrion is a feminine part, because it inherits maternal DNA. I will explain later on, but on the contrary, the cells dependent on energy production by the glycolysis pathway are very masculine. Among them is sperm which carry very few mitochondria as opposed to the ovum.

We carry on our everyday lives while inside of our bodies, both the masculine and feminine components are working together.

We can discover the tips on how to live in a balanced way by exploring the relationship between the two.

An Ovum Matures by Warming It

We can confirm the fact that the mitochondrion is a maternal part by examining functions of the ovum.

When an ovum matures, it is believed that approximately a hundred thousand mitochondria exist in the ovum. Red muscles, the heart and brain where the numbers of mitochondria are significant carry about 4-5 thousand mitochondria. From this comparison alone, we can see that a massive number of mitochondria exist in the matured ovum.

The ovum finishes its cell divisions while in the embryonic development stage where oxygen is limited. So, a woman already has enough ova that she can use in her lifetime when she is born. These ova would be warmed inside of her body. When she reaches around 15 years old, the time when she first starts menstruating, each ovum carries about a hundred thousand mitochondria.

After the first menstruation, women would have their period once a month; the ovulation releases a matured ovum each time. Women reach menopause around 50 years old, so approximately in 35 years, a women uses about 3-4 hundred ova in her lifetime.

On the other hand, sperm contain few mitochondria, so it repeats cell divisions by utilizing the glycolysis pathway. One sperm carries approximately one hundred mitochondria. The cell division of sperm is encouraged because the antiproliferative gene is lacking as only small numbers of mitochondria exist inside of sperm.

The few mitochondria inside of the sperm can enter inside of the ovum at fertilization, but it is broken down in the early stages. You can understand that when a hundred million sperm swim toward one ovum, the woman (ovum) has a stronger position.

Characteristics of ovum and sperm can be explained as the following:

Ovum = Mitochondrial Pathway
Sperm = Glycolysis Pathway

By looking at the difference between the characteristics of reproductive cells, you can understand that the process of having a child and the unification of male and female originated from the union of anaerobic bacteria and aerobic bacteria (mitochondria) from the ancient times.

To summarize, reproduction originated from the union of cells (two organisms) that occurred about 2 billion years ago.

Secrets of the relationship between men and women revealed by comparing the sperm and ovum

Sperm (Male)	Ovum (Female)
Glycolysis Pathway Dominant (Anaerobic Exercise)	**Mitochondrial Pathway Dominant** (Aerobic Exercise)
Cell Divisions in Cool Temperature (sensitive to heat)	**Matures when warmed** (sensitive to cold)
Tendency for shorter life Average life expectancy: 79 years old	**Tendency for longer life** Average life expectancy: 86 years old

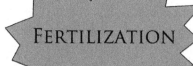

FERTILIZATION

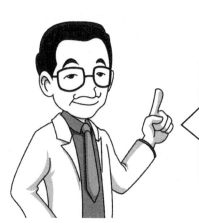

The process in which male and female are attracted to one another, and the fertilization and reproduction of new life, originated from the union of anaerobic bacteria and aerobic bacteria (mitochondria) from the ancient times.

The oxygen dependent aerobic bacteria (female factor) rescued the glycolysis pathway dependent anaerobic bacteria cells (male factor) from their suffering within the increasing levels of toxic oxygen. At the same time, the male factor obtained massive power in return for providing the nutrients to the female factor.

Men need women to survive – the relationship between male and female has been passed on from one generation to the next as it has been done since the ancient times.

In short, mitochondria which have an important role of maintaining our lives depict how women are equipped to protect and nurture children. To leave descendants in the next generation, women utilize men (the glycolysis pathway dependent sperm). In this process, we can glimpse at the origin of the relationship between men and women.

Men are suitable for going out in society and working energetically. To continue to work energetically require the anaerobic state, so men tend to overwork which impose too much stress on their bodies. This could shorten their life expectancy.

During the 60 years period after the end of World War II, the average life expectancy of Japanese people has been extended by approximately 30 years. Japanese men's life expectancy is 79 years old which is not as long as women's life expectancy at 86 years old. 80% of the population of those that are 100 years old and above is also women.

As I mentioned earlier, it is important to note that **women use the energy predominantly produced by the mitochondrial pathway. So, women are biologically suitable for protecting the home and having children. If women work too hard, then the burden of stress imposed on their bodies have greater affect than that of men.**

There have been various opinions on women's advancement in the workplace and society. If we look at this issue purely from the biological standpoint, then women will enter the lifestyle where they will need to depend on the glycolysis pathway, which is a very stressful environment for women's bodies. Stress from overworking can impose a greater effect to women than to men who are biologically more used to using the glycolysis pathway.

If my female readers could take a mental note about this aspect and consider this factor when choosing her work environment, her role and responsibilities at her job, I think it will be helpful for her to maintain a balanced lifestyle.

When she decides to choose a stressful position, then it is fundamentally important for her to keep her body warm. When she keep this in her mind, it will be easier for her to adjust to the workplace and in the society.

Reasons Why Women Turn Beautiful

A secret of women's strength is hidden in her biological connection to the dominant environment of the mitochondrial pathway. I would like to explain this strength from the point of immunology.

The focus point here is the relationship between female hormones and the immune system.

The female hormone (estrogen) is an important substance to form the human body as female. As women reach puberty and the age suitable for marriage, secretion of estrogens increases. At the same time, the dominance of the Parasympathetic Nervous System (PNS) appears.

As I explained in the earlier chapter, PNS becomes dominant when we are relaxed. When our bodies are relaxed, the numbers of lymphocyte increase. This is how the secretion of estrogens increases the immune system.

Also, when the secretion of estrogens increases, women's bodies become curvy and their skin become more youthful and smooth. As a result of the secretion, women obtain attractive bodies.

The process of women turning beautiful correlates with the process of women's bodies preparing for pregnancy and delivering a child.

The natural and more suitable environment for woman's bodies appears between the ages from 20s to 40s. If women live in the lifestyle where the Sympathetic Nervous System (SNS) is dominant, then it imposes a burden on their bodies.

As the tension of SNS continues, numbers of lymphocyte in the blood decrease while the numbers of granulocyte increase. For patients with diseases such as cancer and AIDS, we often observe that numbers of lymphocyte in the blood decreased from 30% to 10% in one month before they passed away.

I have just mentioned the ultimate example, but when women have stressful lives and continue to have the body environment of hypoxia and hypothermia, then female hormones become unbalanced. Women may start to complain about general discomforts and have menstruation problems as a result.

Many women in modern times may have issues with infertility.

This can be caused by the ovum not maturing enough. As the environment of hypoxia and hypothermia continue in women's bodies, women start to have a prolonged ovulation phase as a result.

Drugs that encourage ovulation artificially, such as an ovulation inducing agent does not fundamentally solve the issue of infertility. Since these drugs encourage the environment of hypoxia and hypothermia to continue, there are also potential health concerns by using these drugs.

To overcome the body condition that may result in infertility, it is most important to re-examine the stressful lifestyle which induces a SNS dominant environment in the body.

For women, as you overwork, you tend to get stuck in the state of hypoxia and hypothermia. Such a body environment limits the activities of mitochondria which should be active under normal conditions. As a result, ovulation can be affected and you may lose the natural attractiveness as women.

To talk about the differences as women and men is to learn about our own uniqueness. Such understanding can help us to live the lifestyle in which we can avoid feeling unwell and getting sick. To maximize your own ability and to lead a healthy life for yourself, please note what I explained in this chapter.

Why Are There So Many Women Who Are Sensitive to the Cold?

So far, I explained about how men and women have inherited the distinctive biological characteristics while comparing unique differences between sperm and ovum.

Sperm increases in the glycolysis pathway dominant environment and ovum matures in the mitochondrial pathway dominant environment. Men and women may need to consider what kind of environment is suitable for them, while being mindful about these biological characteristics between male and female.

To repeat what I explained already, sperm repeats cell divisions under cool temperatures. In comparison, ovum matures when it is kept warm.

Regardless of gender, we should all keep our bodies warm in general. For men, it is also important to partially cool their body temperature down, as they have their reproductive organs as external organs. Men become strong by doing so.

Men → Become strong by cooling their body temperature down partially
Women → Mature by keeping their bodies warm

Men need to survive in the stressful environment in the society, and it is important for them to cool down sometimes. On the other hand, if men only live in a warm and a comfy environment, then they are not utilizing the best of their own abilities.

This is also related to the recent issues of sperm count decrease in men.

To encourage the cell division of sperm and continue to live their daily life energetically, it is necessary to modestly work out by utilizing the energy produced via the glycolysis pathway.

Skin also gets thicker and stronger in cooler temperatures because cell divisions are encouraged in such environment. When kids stay home and only play video games, that may lead to health concerns later on.

Men especially need to be creative about how to make full use of the energy they produced via the glycolysis pathway. Using the glycolysis pathway wisely **and not overworking should lead to the full use of men's strength, in other words, to be a man.**

On the other hand, women tend to be more sensitive to the cold than men. You may know the answer to this by now - it is probably because women need to protect the ovum as a biological instinct. To be attentive about keeping a warm temperature is very important for women to maintain the core foundation of the most harmonious balance.

It is essential for women to be careful about not drinking too much cold liquids, and to put on warm clothing when it is cold outside. Also, it is important to be mindful about overtime hours and lack of sleep, as these can create conditions of hypoxia and hypothermia.

For additional information, both before and after the war, the longest life expectancy for women has been reported in the warmest city in Japan, in Okinawa. In contrast, Nagano, the city with a cooler temperature located at a higher altitude reports that they have the longest life expectancy among Japanese men. Where people live does not solely determine the life expectancy of the population, but they are interesting statistics.

You may discover tips for living a healthy life and having prosperity in leaving descendants behind by examining the climates of where you are living now.

Relationship between Cancer Cell Division and Division of the Embryo

We have looked into the difference between men and women in previous sections of this chapter so far. Let's take a look at the fertilization phase now, in which distinctively different men and women are united.

From the fertilization phase and pregnancy to the birth of the child, the glycolysis pathway is the main energy source throughout this process. I am going to explain this in detail by first looking into men who produce sperm.

Testes produce sperm. While the embryo (fetus) is growing inside of the mother's womb, cell divisions have not started yet. By the time the male baby is born, testis goes down to the sac shaped organ called the scrotum, and this is where cell divisions of the sperm start.

The scrotum is an external organ so it maintains a temperature of approximately 5° C (≒ 9° F) lower than the internal body temperature. This environment is an advantageous condition for cell divisions. This 5° C is an important point. If the temperature is lower than this, then both the glycolysis pathway and the mitochondrial pathway may not function properly which can lead to death by hypothermia.

As the boy reaches puberty, the testes increase its capacity dramatically and massive cell divisions occur. When a man ejaculates semen, it can release about one hundred million sperm at one time.

On the other hand, as I mentioned earlier, women already have enough ovum (oocyte) for her lifetime when she is born. The important thing for women is to warm the ovum so that it can mature.

The ovum is produced in the ovary. It matures inside of the ovary. When women start their menstruation cycle, one ovum is pushed into the uterus every month.

When the ovum unites with sperm right after ovulation, it becomes fertilized and leads to pregnancy. However, if the timing is not right, then it does not lead to the fertilization of the ovum.

Women's base body temperature increases soon after the time of ovulation. This is to increase the secretion of female hormones to encourage implantation. By keeping the body temperature warm, women's bodies prepare for pregnancy and the delivery of a baby as well.

Sperm is produced by cell divisions → The Glycolysis Pathway
Ovum matures in the warm temperature → The Mitochondrial Pathway

After these two units are combined and women get pregnant, during the next period of 10 months and 10 days until the birth of the baby, the embryo (fetus) repeats cell divisions by utilizing energy production via the glycolysis pathway.

This may surprise you, but the embryo's process of cell division is very similar to that of cancer cells. As we learned in the earlier chapters, cell divisions occur in the environment of hypoxia and hypothermia.

Of course, the mother's body itself should not fall into hypothermia. When the embryo is implanted in the uterus, the condition of hypothermia is induced by the mother's body reducing the oxygen partial pressure to a quarter of the surrounding environment via the placenta. In this condition, the embryo repeats cell divisions.

In this low oxygen environment, activities of mitochondria slow down. By this, the embryo obtains an ideal condition for cell divisions.

Secret of Timing of People Falling in Love

The embryo (fetus) gradually grows by receiving nutrients and oxygen that the mother consumed via placenta. Also, the embryo excretes wastes and carbon dioxide via the placenta as well.

When we talk about the growth of the embryo (fetus) here, it refers to the cell divisions of the fertilized ovum.

To go into detail, right after the fertilization, the ovum still carries many mitochondria inside, so the cell divisions of the fertilized ovum start slowly.

As two fertilized ovum divide into 4 and then to 8, numbers of the mitochondria in the ovum decrease, and in contrast, the speed of cell divisions increases. After 10 months and 10 days, the speed of cell division reaches its peak. This is how only one fertilized ovum grows into a fetus who can weigh 2000 - 3000 grams (4.4 lb - 6.6 lb).

By this point, the number of mitochondria is so small in the fetus's body, but as soon as the baby cries out and inhales air (oxygen), cell divisions start to slow down. The baby starts to breathe on his/her own, and as the baby is taking in the oxygen, the numbers of mitochondria start to increase.

It is fascinating to see how mother's body controls the environment for the embryo (fetus), creating an advantageous condition for the glycolysis pathway to produce energy, and how the number of mitochondria starts to increase once the baby starts to breathe.

As I mentioned earlier, the speed of cell division reaches its peak while the baby is still in the womb. As the baby enters this world, and the numbers of mitochondria in the body gradually increases, cell divisions in the body continue gradually as well, especially for the heart, brain and red muscle until the person reaches about three years old. As the numbers of cells reach the numbers appropriate for an adult, then the cell divisions stop immediately.

As the old proverb says, "A three year old's soul lasts until the child becomes one hundred years old", tissues and organs developed before the age of three become the foundation of one's life.

Cell divisions continue where the number of mitochondria is limited; for example, the sperm in the testes and skin tissues. As a whole though, the human body gradually depend on the mitochondrial pathway as they grow, and when we reach 20 years old, then we enter the period of the most balanced and harmonious existence.

During this period, men and women become attracted to one another and unite their sperm and ovum by having sexual intercourse. This will lead to a new life being born. And the process of pregnancy to the delivery of the child is repeated again and continues as explained earlier.

This is how a life leaves descendants in the next generation and achieves evolution.

How people fall in love, and how they are attracted to each other and become united, are all parts of the providence of nature which is strongly related to the relationship between the glycolysis pathway and the mitochondrial pathway. Life is still controlled by the natural law which we have inherited from the age of the eukaryote.

As we go through the period of the most balanced and harmonious life and enter the stage of aging, the mitochondrial pathway becomes dominant. People are liberated from their missions of leaving descendants behind and slowly are freed from the need to unite with the other sex. Our life begins with being in the environment where the glycolysis pathway is dominant and ends in the environment where the mitochondrial pathway is dominant.

The mechanism of life we are equipped with is very exquisite, and the core foundations of relationship between men and women are indeed very dramatic.

5 °C (≒ 9 °F) Difference is a Condition for Reproduction

What we talked about in this chapter also apply to other multicellular organisms. It is not exclusive to humans.

The key to reproduction is cell divisions, and the important point is learning how to induce the partial environment of hypoxia and hypothermia. Actually, organisms are very creative in constructing the suitable environment for cell divisions.

We can see this in birds, amphibians, reptiles and fishes.

First, let's take a look at birds. Sperm from the male bird and ovum from the female bird unite by copulation. Then the fertilized ovum is covered by a shell made of minerals and pushed outside of the female body.

To encourage cell divisions for the fertilized eggs, it is necessary to create the condition of hypoxia and hypothermia. Parent birds nest upon fertilized eggs while creating the environment where the temperature is 5 ° C lower than the base body temperature. **Hens' base body temperature is about 42° C (≒ 108 ° F), but eggs are kept under the temperature of 37° C (≒ 99 ° F). This 5 ° C (≒ 9 ° F) difference is the key for creating the state of hypothermia which is perfect for cell divisions.**

When we look at hens' brooding, we think that they are trying to warm the eggs. But in reality, they are inducing the environment of hypothermia, which is 5° C lower than the hens' body temperatures. Combination of the body temperature of hens and air temperature create the difference.Amphibians also push eggs outside of their bodies, but they do not brood like birds. Then, how do they create the condition for cell divisions?

The key to this is the place where they lay their eggs. Amphibians lay eggs by the water. By doing so, they are inducing the 5 ° C difference. They lay eggs during the winter. Eggs hatch in the spring because the spring sun perfectly induces suitable conditions for hatching.

Reptiles often lay eggs on the ground, which is different from amphibians, but the fundamental point of inducing the 5 ° C difference is the same.

For example, sea turtles create the 5 ° C difference by laying eggs in the sand on the beach. Alligators create nests by the water with leaves and weeds, and the 5 ° C difference is made by using the sunlight and the humidity formed by the nest.

Snakes wrap up their eggs with their own bodies to create the 5 ° C difference.

Fishes, like salmon, return to the river of their birth and dig a hole to make a place to lay eggs. They too, create 5 ° C difference by doing so.

If the temperature difference is less than 5 ° C, then the number of mitochondria increases which slows down the cell divisions. Also, if it is more than 5 ° C difference, then the metabolism is blocked which prevents cell divisions.

Life is born in the intricately balanced environment which encourages reproduction via cell divisions.

All multicellular organisms found a way to adapt to the environment and repeat the process of reproduction to leave descendants in the next generation. Both the glycolysis pathway and the mitochondrial pathway co-exist inside of a cell, which reflect the roles of men and women (male and female). The necessity of the reproduction was naturally born.

Why Do Children Hate Green Peppers?

At the end of this chapter, I would like to add a couple things about child development after birth.

Newborns still go through cell divisions so they require solid nutrients. Breastfeeding serves the purpose of effectively supplying the important nutrients to newborns for cell divisions which require the energy from the glycolysis pathway.

As I explained in an earlier chapter, even after the weaning stage, the period of the glycolysis pathway dependency continues a little while so children need to consume foods (glucose).

When the glycolysis pathway becomes dominant, then the children become very active. In general, the SNS become too dominant when people are active. However, children's bodies naturally make the PNS more dominant to balance the environment of their bodies.

Children often hate vegetables like green peppers and carrots, the foods with strong tastes. Actually, when they are still small, their mitochondria are not matured either. Thus the mitochondria which command the detoxification cannot process the polyphenol which is often contained in vegetables with a distinctive taste.

When we tell children to eat these vegetables because they are nutritious, they may refuse to eat them. Actually, this has nothing to do with their temperament, but comes from their instincts. As they grow older, the mitochondria are developed so they will naturally start eating these vegetables. I wanted to mention this - it may reduce some mothers' frustration and stress.

Until the mitochondria become active, the period of childhood continues. As we grow older, our tastes changes and we start to like vegetables with strong tastes. This is an indication that we grow into adulthood and the mitochondria are activated.

As women and men have their distinctive characteristics, children do as well. The law of nature decides all these unique characteristics. To follow the providence of nature means to understand this uniqueness and to live our lives by utilizing it.

If you encounter struggles in your life, then please look at the law of nature and find your divergence. Even in the difference between men and women, its meaning exists.

People think that the relationship between women and men has many mysteries. The relationship between men and women follow the law of nature, and knowing this meaning is the key to a life with happiness.

From Abo Laboratory 5:
Warmth for Women and Cold for Men?

The relationship between men and women have been explored by people in all times and places. However, the origin of it is treated as if it is a mystery. When we go back to the history of evolution, it becomes clear that its origin goes back to the union of cells (the anaerobic bacteria with the glycolysis pathway and the aerobic bacteria with the mitochondrial pathway) that occurred two billion years ago.

All multicellular organisms repeat the union of cells by going through the process of reproduction which unites males and female. The ovum matures in the environment where the mitochondrial pathway is dominant and sperm increases in the environment where the glycolysis pathway is dominant.

This is the key to reveal the reasons why the ovum matures in warm temperatures and the sperm increase in the cool temperatures.

Usually, a man and a woman who fall in love with each other during the "period of the most balanced and harmonious existence (20s - 50s)", which can achieve the unification of sperm and ovum. After the unification of the sperm and ovum, the embryo (fetus) creates an environment where the glycolysis pathway is dominant and the mitochondrial pathway is suppressed. The embryo (fetus) grows by cell divisions in that environment and keeps growing to continue the cycle of life-long inherited since beginning of the biological life on this earth.

Chapter 6: Use of Viscous (Sticky) Blood

Cause of Viscous Hypoxia and Hypothermia

In this chapter, let's learn about matters relating to blood.

A thorough network of blood spreads to all parts of our bodies. Every time the heart beats, blood is carried via this network to the capillaries throughout the body. The capillaries carry blood to 60 trillion cells, which consist of tissues and organs, muscles and nerves.

The role of blood is to deliver nutrients and oxygen we took in via the intestines and the lungs to cells in the body. As I explained in the earlier chapters, these nutrients and oxygen are important fuel for powerhouses (the glycolysis pathway and mitochondrial pathway) within the cells.

Of course, in addition to delivering the fuel to cells, it has a role of carrying wastes and carbon dioxide to outside of our bodies.

Erythrocytes (Red Blood Cells), one of the components of blood are in charge of carrying these elements in and out. Also, white blood cells (WBCs) or immunocytes work within the blood. WBCs have the role as protective troops, guarding our bodies from foreign substances. The number of WBCs is significantly less than the number of erythrocyte (1/660), but nonetheless, WBCs also have an important role in maintaining our body functions.

For example, when I examine the collected blood sample under the microscope, I can see various food scraps and bacteria moving between erythrocytes. One of the WBCs' roles is to process these foreign substances, especially since the macrophage and granulocyte capture them and eat the foreign substances one after another.

When we eat too much, the amount of nutrients in the blood increase and defensive cells become occupied with processing these nutrients. As a consequence, the macrophage become slower in processing bacteria and the immune system weakens.

In addition to over-eating, being under stress on a daily basis can create the condition of hypoxia and hypothermia, which can be problematic to the condition of blood. Blood can become acidic and erythrocytes result in sticking with one another. This condition induces viscous blood which can be harmful to the body.

If the viscosity in the blood continues, cholesterol that was absorbed in the blood becomes acidic. This condition increases the risk of arteriosclerosis. It can create thrombus (blood clots) which may lead to strokes and heart attacks.

On the other hand, when we manage stress well in our daily lives and consequently, our bodies do not enter the state of hypoxia and hypothermia, then the combined erythrocytes separate from one another again and each erythrocyte can move freely. Blood becomes smoother which flows better. Naturally, improved blood flow can carry oxygen, nutrients and wastes in a better, balanced way as well.

Also, if you are mindful about eating modestly, defensive cells do not get occupied with processing nutrients all the time which allows the increase of mitochondria's activities within cells.

The smooth blood is often considered as evidence of a healthy condition. A characteristic of erythrocytes which can stick to one another or separate from one another has a strong connection to this condition.

Is Smooth Blood Flow Healthy?

I would like to note here that describing the blood fluidity as smooth and viscous can create a misunderstanding. It is important to mention here first that smooth blood flow does not necessarily mean a good (healthy) condition and that viscous blood does not always refer to a bad (unhealthy) condition.

Actually, many people have an image of blood as something which keeps flowing, but that is not always true.

For example, if you place a cold towel on your fingertip, then the blood flow on your fingertip stops – it takes no more than one second to stop. A small action like this can stop the flow of blood, which is another characteristic.

Then, what does happen inside of our bodies when the blood flow stops?

To cool down means that it leads to hypothermia, and when peripheral blood flow stops, it can lead to hypoxia. In short, it creates the condition of hypoxia and hypothermia and the blood near the fingertips switches to the glycolysis pathway from the mitochondrial pathway. Of course, once we warm up the fingertip, it switches its energy production back to the mitochondrial pathway again.

Like this example, the speed of blood flow changes or sometimes it stops in accordance with the external environment. Blood is pumped out from the heart to all parts of the body, but at the same time, blood flow is delicately controlled in the peripheral blood vessel.

To sum up, **even for a healthy person, the speed of blood flow** changes in response to the conditions of the external environment – blood sometimes flows smoothly and the other times flows slower due to the increased viscosity of the blood.

It is not so simple to distinguish that the smooth blood is good for you and that the viscous blood is bad. This also is in line with the theme in my book – these conditions are also one of the adaptive responses of our bodies, and it is not something we can label as good or bad.

Both conditions of blood are necessary and that is why these conditions occur. I believe that to think we can become healthy by removing the viscous condition of the blood is a similar concept as thinking "we can treat cancer by removing the cancer cell itself".

I mentioned in my book repeatedly, but let us think again about whether the three major cancer treatments; operation, chemotherapy and radiation therapy, successfully reduced the numbers of cancer patients so far. Let us also ask a question of whether humans have successfully overcome cancer. The answer to these two questions is no - in many countries in the world, cancer is the most deadly disease and the numbers of cancer patients are increasing year after year.

To face these realities, we need to grasp the causes of diseases with flexibility to fully understand the disease. When we do that, it simply leads us to the fact – viscous blood is not a failure in the same way as how cancer cells are not a failure.

Meaning of Viscous Blood

Now, let's look at the reasons why the erythrocytes (RBCs) aggregate with one another and as a consequence, the blood becomes thicker.

I mentioned how the blood flow stops when we place a cold towel onto a fingertip. Similar changes in blood flow occur by different emotions. To provide you with a specific example, please visualize when you get angry. When we examine the peripheral blood of a person who lost his or her cool, it indicates that the blood flow also stops.

In other words, when a person has been under an increasing level of stress on a daily basis, the SNS becomes dominant which leads to the condition of hypoxia and hypothermia. In this environment, erythrocytes (RBCs) combine with one another which result in viscous blood.

In general, all erythrocytes are negatively charged which result in repelling the other erythrocytes. When our bodies are under a stressful environment, the electric charge of each erythrocyte decreases, losing its repelling strength. As a result, erythrocytes start combining with one another.

When we reflect this with human emotions, it is a similar concept to "being ready for a battle".

When animals happen to face predators or external enemies, it is important to prepare well for the battle and have our morale up. As I explained in chapter 3, this preparation requires our body to maintain the environment of hypoxia and hypothermia to utilize the energy from the glycolysis pathway. Also, by increasing the secretion of adrenalin, we prepare our bodies for battle, increasing the level of glucose and blood pressure.

Looking at this condition from the prospective of blood, it needs to avoid bleeding when we battle. If we lose a lot of blood due to an injury, then we will definitely lose the battle and we may die. So, our bodies slow down the blood flow or stop it.

Also, to prepare for a bacterial infection by injuries, our bodies increase the numbers of self-defense force, the WBC, especially the granulocytes.

You may now understand that the origin of the viscous blood. It is one of the wisdoms of our bodies and one of our strategies for survival.

When I say battle, I'm not only referring to a physical fight which involves fisticuffs and kicking.

For example, especially for businessmen, your society may require you to be tough in the business world when you face various issues and problems at your work.

If a person only focuses on having smooth blood flow, you are easy-going, comfortable and non-confrontational. However, the person may have no hope of getting ahead in the business world. It is a nice personality trait, but at the same time, the person may lose an important chance in his/her career.

When people are at a younger age, the glycolysis pathway is dominant in their bodies. It is sometimes necessary during this period of time to hit the accelerator and throw themselves into the battle ground.

In short, **it is important to get things done when it is necessary. For this situation, blood becomes viscous. In other words, viscous blood is an indispensible condition for winning the battle.**

When we think this way, viscous blood has its reasons and wisdom.

It is important to know that viscous blood is caused by the vital response to the external environment which adapts to stress. It is an adaptive response to survive, to protect one's life.

Viscous blood is also our bodies' adaptive response to emergencies

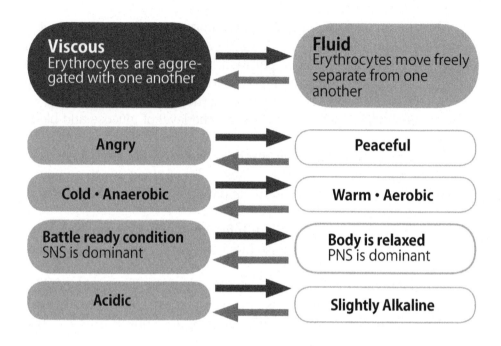

Viscous
Erythrocytes are aggregated with one another

Fluid
Erythrocytes move freely separate from one another

| Angry | Peaceful |

| Cold · Anaerobic | Warm · Aerobic |

| **Battle ready condition** SNS is dominant | **Body is relaxed** PNS is dominant |

| Acidic | Slightly Alkaline |

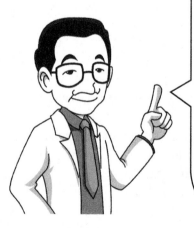

We adapt to the external environment by balancing the viscosity and fluidity in the flow of blood to control our mental and physical conditions. You may have an image of smooth blood flow being healthy, but in some situations, smooth blood flow may not be ideal for our bodies. For instance, when we need to prepare for battle or when we face stressful situations in our lives. Of course, continuing to have viscous blood flow may lead us to various diseases. So, maintaining the balance between these two blood conditions is also important.

Reasons Why the Diameter of the Erythrocyte Is the Same Length as the Capillary

Viscous blood is also wonderful. I realized this fact when I was observing the blood under the microscope.

Erythrocyte is flat shaped and dented in the middle. When they reach the peripheral blood vessel, it awkwardly moves inside of the vessel by being tilted, combining with others or bumping into others.

Then, I realized that the diameter of the capillary is 7.5 mm (micrometers = 0.0075mm). The diameter of the erythrocyte is also 7.5 mm. At the point when the erythrocytes enter the capillary, it becomes harder for the erythrocytes to move smoothly inside of the capillary.

"How come the erythrocytes are moving in such a constricted way?"

It was when I asked this question that I realized the fact I mentioned earlier: "the blood's purpose is not only to flow smoothly".

If the purpose of blood is to flow smoothly, then the diameter of erythrocytes should be smaller than the diameter of the capillary.

In reality, erythrocytes flow inside of the capillary, all cramped up and bumping into one another.

In the experiments of blood flow that I mentioned earlier, we confirmed that the erythrocytes combined with and separated from one another in the matter of a second.

Membranes of the capillary endothelial cells are negatively charged, so the erythrocytes that are also negatively charged do not usually stick to the membranes of the capillary endothelial cells. However, when human bodies are under stress, the membranes lose its charge strength and at last, the erythrocytes stick to the membranes.

Just like this, both fluid blood and viscous blood are being controlled. The key to the blood flow change is stress from the external environment.

When we come across stress, then our bodies need to be conditioned in order to prepare for battle. Blood becomes viscous by erythrocytes being combined. After the body is being released from the preparation for battle, then the blood flows smoothly again.

This is a physiologic function of our bodies. When we talk about the viscous blood as an unhealthy condition and say that it is not good for the body or that it is the cause of disease, then the focus of these discussions may not be on the point.

In any case, I am also surprised by this discovery.

I have achieved various discoveries as an academic researcher so far. However, I discovered the main themes of this book; "cancer is not caused by our bodies' failure" and "blood is not always flowing but sometimes it stops its flow", only after I became 60 years old.

Erythrocytes were controlling the blood flow of capillary!

The diameter of the capillary is 7.5 mm. Also, the diameter of an erythrocyte is 7.5 mm. In this situation, it is hard for the blood to flow smoothly. At the end of veins, erythrocytes are often combined with each other or get separated from one another. By doing this, our bodies control the internal conditions.

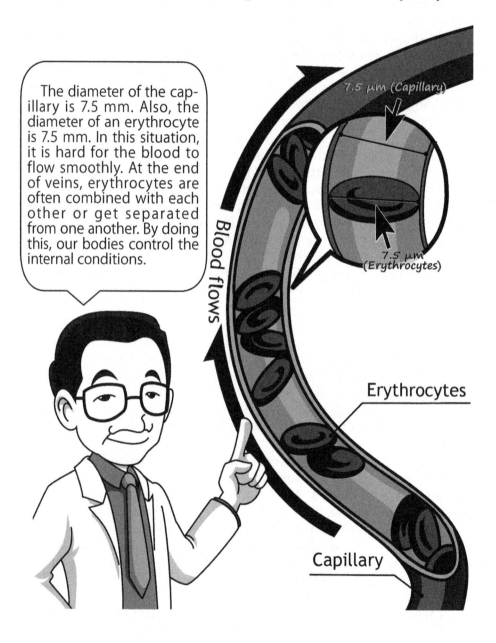

The latter one probably sounds so simple. However, fundamentally understanding this fact can change our approach to the disease dramatically. I am repeating myself again, but remember: Getting sick is not always a bad thing. It has meaning and it happens because it is necessary.

Conditions for Cancer's Spontaneous Remission to Begin

To understand the elaborate control of the blood by the erythrocytes, let me add a couple more important points.

The surface of the erythrocytes, like other cells, is covered by the cell membrane. On the cell membrane, there are a lot of complex carbohydrates (glucide), called the sugar chain are spread out. On the tip of this sugar chain, there is a kind of sugar called sialic acid. It is understood that the sialic acid works as a medium, communicating between the cells, combining them and separating them.

Actually, the erythrocytes contain a significant amount of sialic acid. That is why the erythrocytes can easily combine with one another or separate within the capillary.

Moreover, there is a potential difference between the inside and outside of the cells separated by the cell membrane (membrane potential). Both erythrocytes and capillary have negative electric potentials, so that they are compatible with each other. It also prevents the erythrocytes from combining with the capillary and preventing the blood flow.

These remarkable facts on the control of blood flow can also be confirmed by analyzing the pH level of the blood, determining whether the blood is alkaline or acidic.

Usually, blood is slightly alkaline between pH 7.35-7.45. When the blood becomes viscous by erythrocytes aggregating with one another, the pH level goes down to less than pH7.35 and start to become more acidic. When we assess the pH level of blood from cancer patients, with no exceptions, it shows less than pH 7.30.

Amazing thing is when we start keeping the bodies of cancer patients warm, then the pH level of blood also starts to return to being slightly alkaline. When its pH level increases beyond 7.35, then spontaneous remission of cancer begins. Body regains its strength to cure when viscous blood turns into smooth blood.

Of course, what is important here is a balance. By continuing to keep the body warm, the blood can reach the point where it is too basic which also causes stress to the body. When the pH level reaches to pH7.50

-7.60, then the body is at a thermal crisis. This condition is perfect for remitting cancer cells, but this condition is also at a thin line with going beyond the human body's limitation and losing one's life as well.

It is often helpful to incorporate the stone sauna and hot spring bathing for cancer remission, but please do not forget that balance is very important. If you over-bathe in the stone sauna and hot spring, then it may lead to a thermal crisis or getting a hot flush. It could also lead to a fatal condition so please remember to maintain a balance.

It may surprise you, but the cancer cell can remit due to fevers when we get an infectious disease, because the fever relieves our bodies from the conditions of the hypoxia and hypothermia.

When our body temperature increases, it can not only activate the lymphocyte, but also bring the pH level of the blood back to being slightly alkaline. However, at the same time, we cannot force our bodies to have a high temperature. So, I suggest we use a hot water bottle or a hot bath to keep our body warm to encourage the spontaneous remission of cancer.

Why does Blood Rise Up to the Head?

I have digressed from what I was talking about, but we were talking about how getting angry and getting excited can cause blood to be viscous. It also immediately uses energy from the glycolysis pathway.

By doing so, the body prepare for battle as I have mentioned earlier. Even if this condition is the adaptive response of our bodies to stress, it can be harmful to the body if this condition continues for a long time.

If our bodies are under the battle ready conditions every day and we do not improve the quality of our lifestyles, then it can create a hotbed for canceration. In this sense, how the viscous blood can lead to getting disease may be true.

You can visualize how the erythrocytes collide with each other as how human relationships are depicted in various soap operas. The relationship in soap operas is sticky and that is how viscous the inside of the capillary becomes when the bodies are preparing for battle. It is important for people in this condition to find a peace of mind which can reset our emotions. When we reset, the blood can flow smoothly inside of the capillary again.

For example, we sometimes describe getting angry as "blood rising up to the head". This explains the condition where the flow of blood is gathered in the brain all at once and thus the brain is activated immediately.

When we get excited and the SNS becomes dominant, it leads to hyperpnoea. This increases the circulation volume of blood and blood flows into brain. As you know brain has a plenty of mitochondria, so when it is supplied with oxygen, it ignites at once.

This condition brings the blood flow mainly to the brain, so the other parts of the body are under the condition of hypoxia and hypothermia, utilizing the energy from the glycolysis pathway.

To express your anger, it may be a perfect condition. However, if you are always in this condition, then it imposes a burden on your body. It also can have a negative effect on the balance of the SNS. It increases the pulse and can trigger hypertension (high blood pressure) and hyperglycemia.

Therefore, it is important to be mindful about our bodies when we get angry. If you do become angry, it is important to put your feelings behind you and move on. We call this 'cooling down' – the meaning of this phrase actually has a scientific fact.

Generally, when a person gets angry at other people or becomes annoyed with someone, the feeling of forgiveness naturally follows. As a result, the excess blood flow into the brain is relieved as well. This is actually a natural response of the human body to anger.

However, by living as a human, there always can be bumps in the road and at some points in your life, there may be a time where you get continuously irritated and lose the balance in your lifestyle.

When you get that continuous feeling of irritation and you are not cooling down, please remember to take a walk for a change. By walking, the lower half of your body is stimulated so the unbalanced blood flow rushing into the brain will be resolved. As a result, you will naturally regain your cool demeanor.

This also applies when you are using your brain intensely for studying or at work.

In the old days, there was a philosophers' trail. Philosophers ponder their thoughts so they use their brain a lot, but at the same time, they also walked to relax and to reset their thoughts. A result of doing so can be an 'Aha!' moment when a new idea suddenly appears in a thought.

What Happens When You Walk While Hotheaded

I would like to explain the condition of blood rising up to the head a little further.

When you have the condition where blood rise up to the head, then you may feel as if your eyesight goes completely white momentarily. This is caused by the retinal cell recognizing an increase in the level of oxygen.

It affects not only the eyes, but also the brain, where there is also an increase in the level of oxygen. In this environment, mitochondria overwork in the brain. Consequently, our brain only can focus on one thing. It becomes hard to judge what is good and bad – this condition is what we call "losing it".

People who can lose themselves over seemingly small matters may be under this condition habitually. This also means that they tend to lose their control over their body and soul.

If you are the person who has a tendency to do so, then please make an effort to move on and to control your body and mind. If you lose yourself, as I already mentioned, make sure to take your time to take a walk slowly or do the deep breathing exercises. Making a habit of "cooling down" is helpful.

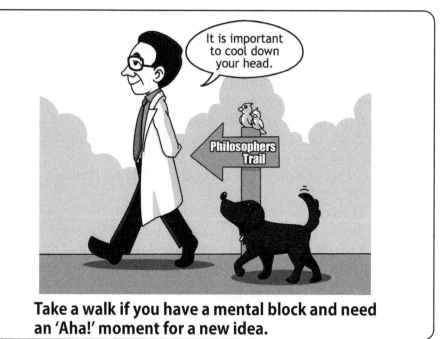

Take a walk if you have a mental block and need an 'Aha!' moment for a new idea.

This practice does not apply only to when you get angry, but it also applies to you when you worry a lot. In both situations, only the brain has a lot of oxygen and other parts of the body lack the oxygen. The pulse increases and hyperpnoea occurs. This condition results in oxygen concentrating in the upper body,

In this case, you should be present and realize that you are under hyperpnoea, and start breathing out slowly and repeat the deep breathing exercises. It may sound so simple, but just by doing this, you will regain your cool.

On the contrary, when something bad happens to you and when you feel emotionally down, then you may feel that your eyesight became completely black.

In this case, both pulse and blood pressure decrease and the circulation of blood slows down as well. As a result of these conditions, the whole body does not have energy. Also, an inadequate amount of oxygen is carried to the retina which leads to the eyesight getting dark.

In this condition, you should lay down for a while so the blood can flow into your brain. By doing this, the retina also gets a supply of oxygen and your eyesight will soon regain the light. You may want to wait until then to take a walk outside for a change of scenery.

Both situations of blood rising up to the head or not rising occur because they are necessary.

When our bodies response to either situations, other conditions such as hypoxia, hypothermia, hyperglycemia or hypertension (high blood pressure) often occur at the same time. The works of SNS as well as the numbers of erythrocytes or WBCs change in accordance with the conditions and environments in our bodies.

Our bodies always try to maintain a balance. Obtaining the wisdom of life starts from understanding this point.

How to Maximize Your Ability in Playing Sports

I mentioned our bodies utilize viscous blood to prepare for battle. In reality, there might be people who have experienced actual battle in a sense – they are athletes.

Athletes are in a way, the people whose profession is to fight in a battle. To be challenged in a game and to win it, it is necessary for them to sharpen the SNS and effectively create the condition of viscous blood with an environment of hypoxia and hypothermia.

In a way, compared to regular people, athletes tend to live with unbalanced body conditions by having viscous blood most of the time for their best performances. It is essential for athletes to balance their body condition though, because if they get stuck in this condition, they may lose mental preparation for the game as a consequence. If they are not prepared mentally, they may not be able to give 100% of the results of their hard practices and training into the game.

The reason why athletes place importance in mental training is because they need to prepare themselves at maximum level where both body and mind is at a perfect balance for the game.

When they achieve this fine balance, then they can show the best of their ability at the game and achieve an unbelievable performance which leads them to win.

For example, Akiko Suzuki, a Japanese figure skater who placed 8th in the Vancouver Winter Olympic in 2010, has been competing in major junior competitions since she was younger. As she advanced in her figure skating career, she struggled to maintain the balance of body and soul. She lost weight significantly due to an eating disorder, and at one point her weight was about 30 kg's (around 66 lbs).

She had struggled to maintain her presence of mind, due to the extreme level of pressure which led to shallow breathing and an increase in her pulse. If we look at her example from the perspective of what I explained in this chapter, her condition was probably caused by the SNS becoming dominant due to the high level of stress.

She spoke about the biggest turning point in her condition when she incorporated Yoga into her exercise routine, which provided her opportunities for deep breathing.

Yoga allowed her to obtain the condition where the PNS is dominant and also she was able to switch back and forth between viscous blood and smooth blood. This resulted in her obtaining the ticket to the Olympics.

First-class athletes have often experienced similar struggles like Ms. Suzuki's, trying to find the fine balance of conditioning and performance.

The reasons why we get excited and often moved by these athletes' performances are not only because that they won a competition, but also because they show us a remarkable performance which is out of the ordinary. They can show us that they achieved the excellent balance by training so hard. This fine balance that the athletes acquire is also a theme for all people, even though each person has their own levels of practices.

When we watch sports, please remember what I explained now and feel the beauty of what the athletes have remarkably achieved for competing. We can also learn from these athletes on how to live our lives which can have a more important meaning for our bodies than focusing just on the winning and losing.

If You Don't Lose Your Cool, You May Grow Senile?

I have suggested you to take a walk so that lower half of your body is stimulated when you feel the blood rise to your head. When you do so, you also need to be mindful about keeping the balance. You will need to adjust yourself case by case. If you keep focusing on training your lower half of your body, then the blood will not flow into the brain. When the brain lacks blood, it means that the brain's functional level decreases.

For example, older people with dementia sometimes stroll and wander around. Lately, an increasing number of older people have a diagnosis of dementia. I think this has a relationship with how people stop stimulating brains by not thinking after they retire.

When people do not think too much, it has a benefit of being released from stress.

However, if you do not exercise your brain or think at all, then you may become senile.

To prevent going senile, it is important to use your upper body. Easy ways to incorporate this is to exercise your fingers.

As you get older, it is also important to use your fingers by perhaps learning piano, calligraphy, knitting and cooking. Please be mindful of using your fingers as often as you can. Please do not only focus on walking every day for your health.

As you use your fingers more, your brain will be comfortably activated and you may realize that you don't forget as much.

On the other hand, if you are a hotheaded type of person at your old age, then it is helpful for you to walk often. This is the same concept as for people who have hypertension (high blood pressure) and hyperglycemia. By walking, you are balancing the blood flow rising up to your brain. Also, please be mindful of resting well at night. Go to sleep early and wake up early. By doing this, you can balance the dominance of the SNS.

I am rather this type of person myself. When I get excited, I raise my voice and my blood pressure shoots up. For a while, I made a habit of taking a walk, but it gets boring after a while to just walk. So, I tried to move my body by taking the garbage out or cleaning outside and around the house.

Also, I usually go to sleep around 9 o'clock at night. I try to be mindful of making the PNS dominant by getting enough sleep.

People in the modern times tend to have a lack of exercise. It is important for each of us to assess our own characteristics and living environment and customize our own ways of keeping the balance between upper and lower parts of our bodies.

When I say exercising, I do not mean that you must go to the fitness club and train until you are exhausted. You don't need to get stressed out by exercising too hard. The secret of maintaining youth and obtaining good health is to discover an exercising method which suits your ability and interest and continue.

Please find something that you can have fun in. Once you find it, try it out and continue exercising.

The Strategy of Our Body's Response to Stress

Our bodies survive by controlling our emotions, and keeping a balance between viscous blood and smooth blood. The reasons why we need to learn how to control our emotions are because humans are homoeothermic animals. At the end of this chapter, let's go over this point quickly.

Homoeothermic animals can change body temperatures on their own. For them, it is necessary to control the body temperature by moving around or hibernating, so that the temperature will be not too high or too low.

Especially for humans, the harmonious balance between the glycolysis pathway and the mitochondrial pathway is needed. We need to use instantaneous force and endurance in a balanced way, as well as need to maintain the intricate condition in our bodies.

Both viscous blood and smooth blood are parts of the intricate condition in our bodies.

Poikilothermal animals whose temperatures change in accordance with the external temperature, can only adapt to the external temperature by changing the places they live. If the environmental conditions on the earth continue to change due to the global warming, these animals may only have a limited range of places to go to and eventually, they'll become extinct in the future.

On the contrary, humans are homeothermal animals, so we can change the way we live by our own wills. In this sense, we are connected to the external environment in a more subjective way.

When you get sick and you realize that your unbalanced lifestyle has caused the sickness, stop hanging on to medical treatments just because you can avoid unpleasant symptoms by doing so. Also, by being obsessed with staying healthy and being scared and stiff about getting diseases, people can derail from the path for a balanced lifestyle too.

As I explained so far, getting sick is a precious chance. It is a chance to realize that you have lost the balance in your body.

Please listen to the signals of your body, such as viscous blood – your body is trying to adapt to the external stress and wisely informing you that you are losing balance.

We, humans, are not only able to be healthy, but also are able to get sick and feel unwell – we live in a perfectly balanced world.

Let's make full use of each of our abilities, by understanding that the viscous blood too has its purpose. If you get tired, then take a good rest so that you can once again have smooth blood flow.

From Abo Laboratory 6:
Viscous Blood is Needed At Times

When our bodies are under the condition of the hypoxia and hypothermia due to the stress, erythrocytes aggregate one another and the blood becomes viscous. People have perceived the condition of the viscous blood as evidence of an unhealthy condition. But we need to look at the condition as a bigger picture.

Viscous blood is formed by our bodies in response to external stress to create a battle ready environment. It is a physiological adaptive response.

As I explained, evidence of that is the fact that the diameter of the capillary is the same diameter as an erythrocyte's. By getting angry and blood rushing up to your brain, erythrocytes at the end of the capillary start to aggregate with one another and the blood become viscous.

In this way, our bodies can face the emergency by hitting the accelerator utilizing the instantaneous force produced by the glycolysis pathway.

Of course, after you worked while using the full acceleration, it is important to take a good rest. Balancing between having the viscous blood and the smooth blood is intricate, but necessary. It is important that we do not only praise about having smooth blood, but also commend us on having viscous blood once in a while. Having viscous blood means we are working hard and pushing our limits.

Chapter 7: Reasons Why Doctors Rely on Medicine

Why Do Patients Increase as the Number of Doctors Increases?

From what is shown of the three conventional treatments, modern medicine offers surgical operation, chemotherapy and radiation therapy as core treatment options for cancer patients. A few doctors may offer their patients with alternative treatment options other than the use of these methods, but the number of these doctors is still small.

At the receiving end, many patients also commonly accept these treatments because many people accept the concept that "surgery and drugs treat sickness".

There is no problem if patients effectively recover from sickness and serious diseases by receiving these treatments. In reality, patients' health may become worse in some cases as I have repeatedly mentioned in this book.

In fact, about 30 years ago in Japan, the numbers of deaths by cancer were about 130,000 people per year. The numbers of doctors back then were approximately 130,000 as well.

Now the numbers of doctors are approaching about 300,000, and the numbers of deaths from cancer are now more than 300,000 a year.

What I would like to mention now is not about whether modern medicine has improved from the past, but about a much deeper concept which concerns the philosophy of viewing life.

The numbers of sick patients keep increasing despite the fact that modern medicine has dramatically improved. Looking at the sickness as evil as a starting point, and focusing on the removal of diseases when the patients are treated, could be causes of this increase.

When we look at the sickness from a different point of view and start accepting the fact that getting sick is the adaptive response of our bodies, we need to consider alternate ways of treating sickness. You may also clearly realize how modern medicine has continued to treat these conditions in a way that has derailed from the fundamental understanding of sickness.

The main concern is how dependent modern medicine became on drugs. When we go to the hospital, doctors prescribe medications even though the symptoms themselves are not so serious.

Also, it is easy for us to go to the pharmacy and purchase medicines. So, many people naturally accept the concept, "when we get sick, we take medicine".

Various medical symptoms can be temporarily improved by tak-

126

ing medications. However, fundamental causes of diseases or physical conditions are not completely cured by medicine. As becoming stressed, having emotional upsets, overworking and having lack of sleep are not improved by the medications, the causes of diseases, the state of hypothermia and hypoxia would continue.

Taking medications will not allow us to truly recover. If the symptoms continue because the fundamental causes are not taken care of, people continue to get sick, and they may continue to be dependent on the medicine.

As these symptoms continue, people go to hospitals again and various tests are done on them. New drugs would be prescribed and as these cycles continue, patients may develop serious diseases such as cancer and end up receiving surgery or chemotherapy. So far, I have explained the problems of the current treatment options that modern medicine can offer. Now, I would like to look at how effective other treatment options can be in treating sickness.

Treatment options which do not use medications can be found in many alternative medicines. Many of these alternative medicines place importance in balancing diets and exercise.

Many people may not be sure which diet they should choose as there are many different diet methods that are currently available.

Before we look into diet and exercise, we should first look at the reasons why drug dependent medical treatments began in the first place.

If a balanced diet is indeed effective, then how come it was not incorporated into the medical treatment in the past? I should analyze this issue first.

Let's go back to Dr. Otto Warburg, the German biochemist I introduced in the Chapter 1. To answer these questions, there are many clues that Dr. Warburg left behind in his research during his time in the early 20th Century.

I would like to follow his research again, so we can identify the issues one by one which prevented modern medicine from becoming nondependent on medications.

Why are Diseases Not Cured as Medical Technology Advances?

Dr. Otto Warburg is a pioneer in decoding the mechanism of energy productions within cells which I also have mentioned throughout this book.

His research revealed mainly about the mechanism of the glycolysis pathway. During his research, he made a very interesting discovery that "the cancer cell obtains energy from the glycolysis pathway (fermentation) even in the environment where oxygen is present".

This was a great discovery. The characteristic of the cancer cell is that it repeats cell divisions utilizing the energy produced by the glycolysis pathway. Cancer cells do this even in the environment where oxygen is available. When oxygen is available, cancer cells have options to utilize energy produced by the mitochondrial pathway, but these cells barely use energy from the mitochondrial pathway.

In other words, cancer cells are cells which can barely utilize the mitochondrial pathway which often suppress cell divisions as the speed of cell divisions increases. Energy productions of cancer cells are mainly fueled by the glycolysis pathway.

Dr. Warburg thought that this characteristic of cancer cells was the key to finding cancer treatments. He continued his research, but it was at a time when we started to gain understanding about the human gene, and it became commonly accepted that the cause of cancer was the mutation of the gene caused by carcinogens.

In this sense, Dr. Warburg's theory can be considered as an old theory which was not spotlighted in the field of modern medicine. However, it does not mean that what Dr. Warburg noted was incorrect. As I explained already in Chapter 1, the mutation of a gene may lead to the development of cancer cells, but this understanding may not lead to the appropriate treatment options for cancer patients.

For example, inhaling exhaust fumes is said to cause cancer, but moving to a rural area does not necessarily lead to the spontaneous remission of cancer.

Avoiding carcinogens does not necessarily help cure cancer. Even though we now identified 'what we can consider as some causes of cancer', we still depend on symptomatic treatment to treat cancer in the field of medicine.

As a result, surgery, use of chemotherapy and radiation therapy was established as the three conventional cancer treatments.

This applied to other diseases as well. The detail studies of genes or functions of mitochondria have advanced. Since these studies are very interesting, the curiosities encourage such advancement. However, looking in detail often let us forget to understand life as a bigger picture, like when we see trees but not the forest.

It is wonderful that various researches have advanced, but it does not necessarily mean that they all provide cures to diseases. As a result, clinicians now depend on symptomatic treatments. Consequently, the field of medicine became dependent on medications. This led to undermining the importance of spending time with patients to cheer them up or of utilizing traditional medicine. As time passed by, it became common medical practice that the diagnosis is often reached by the result of blood tests, even without the use of a stethoscope.

Needless to say, modern medical practice is far from truly curing the cancer. This explains how diseases are not cured even though the medical technology has advanced.

Can Avoiding Carcinogens Prevent Cancer?

So far, I explained how the contradiction of modern medicine came about.

To review once more, it is rare that cancer is caused by external factors such as by carcinogens. When our bodies are in the state of hypothermia and hypoxia due to having stress in our daily lives, the glycolysis pathway is stimulated and thus can result in having cancer.

In other words, it means that the condition of hypothermia, hypoxia and hyperglycemia created by stress matches the conditions where the cancer cell can thrive. So, **as long as people continue to live the lifestyle which mainly utilizes energy from the glycolysis pathway, cancer cells may continue to proliferate. Eventually, the capacities of antioxidants and immunocytes cannot keep up with the handling of cancer cells within our bodies.**

Cells become cancer cells to adapt to the internal body environment which is abnormal. When we understand this, then the methods of dealing with the symptoms are naturally revealed. As we change our internal body environment to the conditions where cancer cells can hardly survive, then the body will adapt to the new condition. By doing so, the spontaneous remission of cancer cells may occur naturally. Cancer cells may stop proliferating, even though we do not remove or try to treat the cancer.

Modern medicine does not recognize this simple logic, but instead labels cancer cells as "failed cells" caused by the mutation of genes. As a result, surgery, chemotherapy and radiation therapy are used to tackle the cancer cells.

Many doctors and researchers noticed the importance of the "Warburg Effect", but they could not reach the understanding that "many diseases are adaptive response of our bodies to stress". Thus, they could not connect the "Warburg Effect" with effective cancer treatment. This also added to the reason why people now commonly think that external factors such as carcinogens are the source of canceration.

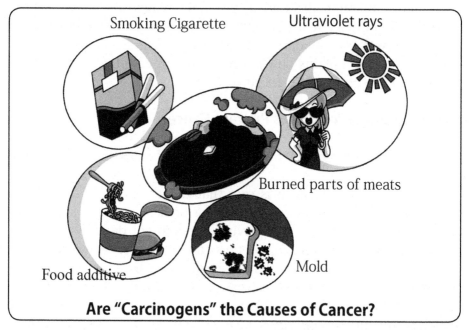

Smoking Cigarette   Ultraviolet rays

Burned parts of meats

Food additive   Mold

Are "Carcinogens" the Causes of Cancer?

In fact, Dr. Warburg himself also had consciously noted that carcinogens could cause cancer, and he even feared the carcinogens while he had an eye on the knowledge that cancer cells proliferate through the glycolysis pathway.

He did not eat any bread sold at the store stating that it was bleached, and selected vegetables that were not grown with chemical fertilizer. He also kept a distance from attending academic conferences and seminars because he disliked inhaling exhaust fumes. His all natural, healthy lifestyle may surprise people in the modern day.

In reality, Dr. Warburg survived until he was 86 years old, and he might have thought that his practice of avoiding carcinogens were correct.

However, as I explained already, thinking that he did not get cancer because he kept a distance from carcinogens does not leave the realm of the imagination. It also does not have any direct connection with the

Warburg Effect.

Canceration by carcinogens can occur at a certain level of frequency. Even if people are attentive about avoiding carcinogens, if they are not prepared for dealing with the stress, then there is a good chance that people can still get cancer.

On the other hand, when people can see through that the main cause of cancer is the conditions of hypothermia and hypoxia caused by stress, then it leads to choosing the effective medical treatment as well.

By grasping the living environments of patients, and teaching them how they can leave the lifestyles in which their body temperatures become lower and they lack in having enough oxygen, then doctors can lead patients to achieve a balance in utilizing both the glycolysis pathway and the mitochondrial pathway.

If we start implementing this, then we may not need to rely heavily on the three conventional cancer treatments.

Also by this, patients can become free from the harmful side effects that come with chemotherapy and radiation therapy, and it may increase the survival rate of cancer patients.

I do not disagree with all the treatments that modern medicine offer, but the treatments options for patients may change if people start to understand what mainly causes cancer.

By understanding the true meaning of the Warburg Effect, cancer can turn into one of the common curable diseases.

Is Cancer a "Renegade Cell"?

Let's follow the flow of what happened in the medical world after Dr. Warburg's time.

Modern medicine achieved two major breakthrough discoveries after Warburg's time, even though researchers were still unable to connect Warburg's discovery to effective cancer treatments.

One of the discoveries was "the endosymbiotic theory", which was advocated by Dr. Lynn Margulis, an American biologist in 1967. About 20 years after Warburg's time, the theory that explained "the powerhouse mitochondria within our cells evolved from external parasitic aerobic bacteria" was mentioned for the first time. I have already explained certain details of this process, but this theory clarified that the mitochondria was an aerobic bacteria, and revealed the clear difference between the aerobic mitochondrial pathway and the anaerobic glycolysis pathway respectively. Dr. Margulis' theory became the foundation of my discovery which revealed the causes of cancer later on.

In other words, in Dr. Warburg's time, it was difficult for researchers to decode the process of canceration or the mechanism of life itself, even though researchers could see the adaptive response of human bodies when the cancer cells repeat cell divisions of cells by utilizing the glycolysis pathway.

In science, accumulation of discoveries due to predecessors stimulates new ideas and pushes open new doors to the world. I often realize that one researcher cannot work alone in this field.

Another discovery was made by an American biologist, Dr. Robert Weinberg and his colleagues.

They studied oncogenes and tumor suppressor genes. Dr. Weinberg was concerned that a proto-oncogene is carried in the nucleus of a cell .When exposed to carcinogens and altered by mutation, it becomes an oncogene, which is a gene that has the potential to wreak havoc in almost every part of the human body (cause cancer). At the same time, a tumor suppressor gene also exists in a cell and these genes suppress tumor formation. Therefore, cancer will not strike us immediately.

When the speed of divisions of the oncogene increases or the strength of the tumor suppressor gene weakens, there can be an issue with either the acceleration or with breaking, meaning that the body environment can result in the advancement of canceration.

Dr. Weinberg's research became the foundation for cancer treatment today, and has its importance in the field. However, it might have not reached its core since his research sees cancer cells as abnormal cells.

As I explained so far, cancer cells are not "abnormal", but are born in the conditions of hypothermia and hypoxia. True characters of cancer cells are revealed when we start our understanding from the perspective that the canceration is an adaptive response to overcome an emergency.

Dr. Weinberg calls cancer the "one renegade cell". His research could not approach the relationship between condition of hypothermia and hypoxia and cancer cells. As long as the adaptive response is labeled as renegade, it may not be able to cure the cancer.

Unfortunately, if we continue to use Dr. Weinberg's research as the foundation for cancer treatment, incurable treatment methods used in modern medicine may continue on to the future. This might be the reality of modern medicine.

Should We Treat the Cancer of Elderly Patients?

Separately from the common understanding that the cancer is a failure of the body, the understanding of "cancer is caused by aging" has widely been discussed recently.

In Japan, Dr. Keiichi Nakagawa, a director in radiation oncology has been speaking about this theory. When we take works of the glycolysis pathway and the mitochondrial pathway into consideration, then this theory cannot also be said to be true. Because as people age, the glycolysis pathway naturally becomes less dominant, and it is natural that the cancer does not proliferate so much.

It is well known that when doctors conduct an autopsy of an elderly person who died of natural causes, doctors discover many small cancers. However, these cancers are not life threatening, so they are usually not the direct causes of death. **When an elderly person get a cancer, it is often better not to treat it.**

In the old days, doctors understood this from experiences. So, there was an unspoken understanding of "do not aggressively treat elderly patients". In modern days, there is no understanding like this. There are many cases where doctors perform surgery on elderly patients who are over 80 years old.

As I explained in Chapter 4, **people who led stressful lifestyles and used the energy from the glycolysis pathway dominantly during the time when humans have the most balanced and harmonious existence tend to have cancer. The most balanced and harmonious time is between the age 20s and 50s. Without understanding this, the doctors can continue to administer anti-cancer drugs in an attempt to tackle cancer cells. Result of such practices can rather hasten patients' lives.**

It is my opinion that modern medicine can worsen the cancer by doing too much, and as a consequence, it made cancer into a complicated and difficult disease.

Some people reason by looking at the increase of cancer patients among elderly populations in Japan that "Japan has the higher death rate by cancer, because Japan is the country of the most longevity". This kind of reasoning is not even logical.

The higher death rate by cancer is rooted in the modern medicine's failure to appropriately grasp the causes of cancer. If we understand the contradictions we explained so far, both the numbers of patients who get cancer as well as those persons who die of cancer may decrease.

If we do not recognize such contradictions and do not make any modification in the current practice of tackling cancer cells, then cancer will not be cured even though medical technology becomes more highly developed.

As we reveal the true identity of cancer, we see that the canceration is not a mystery, but that cancer is rather a simple disease.

The process of the oncogene growth is based on various factors and varies from one person to another, but cancer is not the disease we need to fear. We do not need to worry too much about cancer and you will naturally know how to get along well with cancer.

I, myself, try to accommodate private telephone consultations as much as I can, but I do not often refer cancer patients to doctors. I want them to understand what a cancer-free lifestyle is and that "to heal their bodies on their own" is the foundation for a cure.

Even for those patients who have been seeing doctors have ways to cope with the situation.

It is important for them to first face the lifestyle of overworking and of having worries and to try to change such a lifestyle on their own.

I will introduce in Chapter 9 "8 Rules for Staying Away from Cancer". I recommend you to refer to them and incorporate them in your daily life.

Reasons Why Dietary Therapy is Effective to Cancer

I would like to return to Dr. Warburg's research. I mentioned earlier that he feared the oncogene and he followed a strict natural diet. There is actually a doctor who inherited this idea and developed it.

His name is Dr. Max Gerson (1881-1959), a German doctor (emigrated to the U.S. later) who is considered to be a founder of dietary therapy for cancer patients.

The dietary therapy that he founded is called the Gerson Therapy, which is mainly based on the intake of fresh vegetables and fruit juices, while avoiding intakes of natrium (sodium) and animal proteins such as meats. This is the originator of various dietary therapies practiced today.

A devotee of Dr. Warburg, Dr. Gerson, came up with his dietary therapy by noting the point that "the cause of cancer might be from dietary habits of westerners who eat a lot of preserved meats with salts".

It is true when we over-eat meats, they wear down the lining of intestines. This can lead to the lack of oxygen which causes cancer. It is necessary to cut our natrium intake to maintain the normal balance between the natrium and kalium (potassium) in the inside and outside of cells.

When there is more natrium in the outer cell and more kalium in the inside of cell, the mineral balance within the cells in our bodies is balanced. However, when we have an over-intake of natrium, the balance weakens and the metabolism in the cells may weaken.

Balance between natrium and kalium is being controlled by the energy produced by the mitochondrial pathway, so if there is more natrium present, then it burdens the mitochondrial pathway as well.

People in the modern day era have a tendency to take in more natrium, and tend not to eat enough vegetables and fruits. These eating habits can indeed create conditions for the division of cancer cells.

The flipside of this is **eating no meat or natrium (salt) but more vegetables and fruits can weaken the works of the glycolysis pathway and be effective in stimulating the mitochondrial pathway. Dietary therapy works because it grasps well the unique characteristics of the cancer cell.**

Therefore, there are still many practitioners of dietary therapy in the modern day, including the Gerson Therapy. During the time of Dr. Gerson, many anti-cancer drugs were also rapidly developed. There were many people who felt resistant to the Garson's dietary therapy method which explained to people that cancers would be cured by improving what people ate. Many doctors did not support his idea and ignored it. In the Gerson Therapy, people could find many clues and hints to cure cancers, but instead of pursuing these clues, modern medicine has chosen to pursue the symptomatic treatment, the method of 'tackling cancer with chemotherapy".

As a result of this, modern medicine became distant from the fundamental truth of all biological life.

Basis for the U.S. Government's Recommendations

It is especially important to note among Dr. Gerson's discoveries that he found causes of cancer in our daily diet. As modern medicine ignored this, it was not widely utilized for a long time. Later on, various methods of dietary therapies following Dr. Gerson's discovery were introduced, and some doctors began to incorporate dietary therapy for patients as part of their cancer treatment. As dietary therapy became recognized, traditional Japanese foods started to receive some attention.

In 1978, the U.S. senator, George McGovern and his colleagues in the Senate Select Committee on Nutrition and Human Needs, compiled a report on foods and health (the McGovern Report) and recommended the "Dietary Goals for the U.S.", explaining that a "daily diet with a large intake of animal proteins like meats can induce cancer", which was a similar concept to the Gerson Therapy. This report became a milestone for the U.S. government to improve the dietary measures for U.S. citizens.

After they reported that many people found that "it is most ideal to eat traditional Japanese foods which consisted of unrefined grains, vegetables and fishes". Macrobiotic, a healthy dietary method, introduced first in Japan became popular in the U.S. and in Europe, which fueled the popularity of Japanese foods.

Parallel to the public recognition of the Macrobiotic diet, dietary therapy methods, such as the fasting diet founded by Dr. Mitsuo Koda, gradually became popular in Japan. Founder of natural medicine, Dr. Keiichi Morishita, who came up with the dietary therapy for cancer treatment is also a part of this movement.

Japanese doctors, such as Dr. Yoshihiko Hoshino and Dr. Takaho Watayo, inherited the Gerson Therapy and they utilized it in the clinical forefront of cancer treatment while making some appropriate modifications.

What is common in these dietary therapies is that eating less meat and more vegetables can lead to the cure of cancer. As I mentioned in the part where I explained about the Gerson Therapy, these dietary therapies provide some breaks for the glycolysis pathway and suppress the divisions of cancer cells.

Of course, the glycolysis pathway has its role in our body functions, so I am not saying that the glycolysis pathway is bad.

As I explained so far, we maintain the daily balance of our health by keeping the balance between the glycolysis pathway and the mitochondrial pathway. Cancer is indeed led by the imbalance and energy dependency on the glycolysis pathway, but this does not mean we should not utilize the glycolysis pathway for energy productions.

Especially, during the period between the age 20s and 50s when we have the most balanced and harmonious existence, we use both the glycolysis pathway and the mitochondrial pathway in a balanced way. If we try to shut down the glycolysis pathway, it needs time for our bodies to get used to this condition. We may feel weary as a result. On the other hand, it is important to overcome this weariness for the dietary therapy to be effective.

The reason why dietary therapies have been inherited since the times of Dr. Warburg and Dr. Gerson, and have many practitioners of these methods even today, is because modern medicine has failed to demonstrate a true cure to various diseases.

It is important to acknowledge the effectiveness of the field like dietary therapy to build the medical treatment that can truly cure various diseases, so we can depart from the medication dependent conventional medicine. Of course, for our bodies, co-existence with the glycolysis pathway is also necessary, so these therapies can perhaps be extreme in the therapeutic sense.

Mechanism of Vitamin C Weakening Cancer Cells

The popular alternative therapy for cancer treatments is not only dietary therapy. In recent years, a unique treatment method called massive Vitamin C infusion therapy has attracted some attention.

The high doses Vitamin C therapy is as its name indicates, is to have doctors administer a large quantity of Vitamin C to cancer patients via drip infusion.

It is known that two times Noble Prize recipient, Dr. Linus Pauling, came up with this method. It is a treatment method which does not fit in the common treatment methods offered by the modern medicine. This simple method rendered positive results - many clinical cases of preventing the development of cancer by this therapy are reported. In 2005, even authoritative organizations of the U.S., such as the National Institutes of Health, reported that this therapy is effective.

In this method, it is said that there is hardly any side effects observed, and when used with chemotherapy, the side-effect of the chemotherapy can be reduced to a minimum. It is said about 10,000 medical doctors in the U.S. have incorporated this treatment method clinically to treat their cancer patients.

This positive effect of preventing the development of cancer by a high dosage of Vitamin C can be explained by the characteristics of cancer cells. As I have explained in my previous chapters, the cancer cells predominantly use the energy produced in the glycolysis pathway.

Vitamin C is processed when glucose from foods are absorbed into cells. However, after the Vitamin C is used, it gets oxidized and requires further processing in the mitochondria with in human cells. Cancer cells only have small numbers of mitochondria within the cells. So, cancer cells have a hard time processing the oxidized Vitamin C.

Thus, when doctors continue to infuse high dosages of Vitamin C, oxides are accumulated only in the cancer cells. As a result, by using this method, we can selectively kill off cancer cells while not harming the other cells. This method does not take the mechanism of cancer cell development into consideration, so it is not always effective. You might have discovered that this high dose Vitamin C infusion therapy for cancer patients sophisticatedly applied the Warburg Effect, too.

Also, the Position Emission Tomography (PET) scan used in the cancer test applied the Warburg Effect as well. PET is a test that intravenously administers a tracer similar to glucose into a vein and determines the positions and sizes of cancer by observing where much of the glucose-like tracer is collected in specific organs or tissues by a specialized camera.

Cancer cells use energy predominantly produced by the glycolysis pathway for cell divisions, so they love glucose. When glucose is infused into the body, then the cancer cells naturally collect the glucose-like tracer. The difference between the cancer cells and normal cells then become obvious.

Since the **over intake of sugar (glucose) can encourage the canceration of cells, it is understandable that many dietary therapy limits glucose intake. Many foods that people in the modern day love to eat, such as meats, sugar and salty foods have the tendency to induce an environment in our bodies where cancer cells can develop.**

How to Evaluate Alternative Medicine

This is a separate stream of movement from the Warburg theory, but after the 1980s, holistic therapy has emerged partially from attempts to connect dots between medical research and clinical fields, which the modern medicine has struggled to achieve. Holistic therapy considers the entire body as a whole life.

The word holistic comes from a Greek word holos, from which the English words whole, health and holy derived.

You can get a sense from these words, but holistic therapy aims to increase the strength of the immune system and spontaneous cure by organically understanding the functions of the body as a whole. Traditional medicines from the East, such as Yoga, Qi Gong and traditional Chinese herbal medicines are part of the holistic therapy.

Traditional Indian medicine, Ayurveda, is also one of the holistic therapies. The therapies I mentioned earlier, dietary therapy or various manual therapies such as shiatsu or massage therapy are also included. Other holistic therapies are aroma therapy, psycho therapy and music therapy, which covers various methods.

These therapies are called alternative medicine, because all these treatment methods are alternative to conventional medicine. These therapies are on the opposite side of spectrum from modern medicine which focuses on removing the individual symptoms or suppressing the symptoms by medications. I will not go over the details of each practice of alternative medicine, but **the ones that are proven to be effective are therapies which lead our bodies to flee from the conditions of hypothermia and hypoxia.**

If you have fundamental understanding that "Diseases (cancer) are not always bad things, it is just an adaptive response of our bodies reacting to the hypothermia and hypoxia caused by stress", then you may discover the meaning of keeping the body warm, balancing the ANS by maintaining the dominance of PNS, or releasing the body from the glycolysis pathway dominant energy productions and utilizing energy from the mitochondrial pathway more. All of these alternative medicines often achieve these purposes.

In modern medicine, we measure the body temperature of patients, too. However, doctors do not do this to observe the hypothermia itself, but to check whether patients have a fever or not.

When we reflect this practice on the natural laws of life, then it is apparent that modern medicine may not be able to offer truly an effective cure to the various diseases.

I do not mean it is better to replace modern medicine with holistic alternative medicine. The alternative medicine is going through a transitional period now, and does not completely grasp the meaning of the laws of life (adaptive response under the conditions of hypothermia and hypoxia), either.

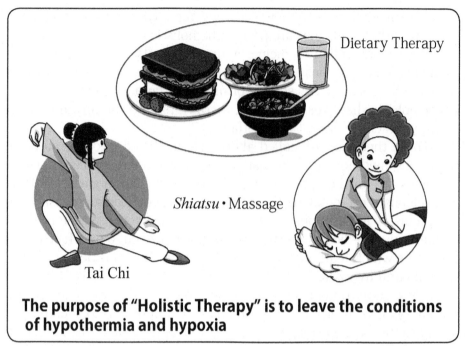

Dietary Therapy

Shiatsu • Massage

Tai Chi

The purpose of "Holistic Therapy" is to leave the conditions of hypothermia and hypoxia

For example, when we take a look at dietary therapy, eating is certainly an important part of our lives. However, eating is not everything. The main concern is how to pay attention to stress. Improving the daily diet may be secondary.

If we do not pay attention to this point, we may not feel the effectiveness, even if we practice dietary therapy. If we do not take care of stress, then the symptoms can get worse. Some of the masters who practice dietary therapy have passed away from diseases even before they reach the average age of life expectancy. This may be because they might have not paid enough attention to reduce stress.

It is the most important to question the meaning of stress and correct the imbalance in the lifestyle that you have led so far. It may be safe to understand that the cancer is often caused by stress, and that when people do not eat foods in a balanced way, then it will lead to canceration.

Recommendations for Evaluating Cancer Treatment

So far, I have touched upon the negative side of dietary therapy, but I do not mean to take the importance of the daily diet lightly.

This can also be said of all holistic therapies, but I believe that each alternative therapy took a big step forward when it denied and questioned the use of anti-cancer drugs.

For example, a Japanese doctor who specializes in radiology, Dr. Makoto Kondo wrote a bestselling book called "Dear Patients, Don't Fight Cancer". He achieved a big step forward when he clearly argued that "anti-cancer drugs are ineffective" to the public.

His theory derailed from the natural laws of life when he argues that radiology, his specialty, is safe. As you know, radiology aims to remove cancer cells so even if radiology itself is safe, the treatment method follows the basic belief that the "bad thing should be removed".

The practice of tackling the cancer cells which are part of the human bodies, lack understanding that cancer cells can have spontaneous remissions. Without this understanding, doctors may not be able to keep patients positive and encourage the spontaneous cure.

Also, radiology decreases the numbers of lymphocytes. Patients may lose strength by that and it may lead to regression of their spontaneous cure.

On the other hand, Dr. Hoshino and Dr. Watayo whom I mentioned in this chapter raised questions to not only the use of anti-cancer treatments, but also to all the three conventional cancer treatments when they followed the Gerson Therapy. Many doctors, who incorporate dietary therapy in treating their patients, probably have this idea when they face patients every day.

This is a good big step forward – but I am afraid that the importance of the daily diet is emphasized too much, because this can lead to other issues as well.

What is most important is "leaving the conditions of hypothermia and hypoxia" and changing the stressful lifestyles. Changing the daily diet alone may not be effective in recovering from the cancer.

In reality, the rate of curing cancer increase when cancer patients switch from conventional therapy to a dietary therapy. However, its results do not indicate dominating effectiveness. This may be because we are paying too much attention to incorporating the knowledge of nutritional science into the field of medicine, but not paying enough attention to the meaning of stress imposed on our bodies in our daily lives.

I would like to explain this issue in detail in the next chapter where I will comprehensively analyze the modern day nutritional science.

Anyhow, you will be able to evaluate the positions and effectiveness of the treatments or self-care practices you have been or you are receiving by seeing these treatments from the standpoint of "leaving the conditions of hypothermia and hypoxia".

You may use this concept when you search for doctors, but what is more important is to understand that having diseases is closely connected to your own lifestyle.

I do not entirely deny modern medicine. However, I argue that sickness should be "self-cured". Before you hold tight onto something else, please take a moment to re-examine your lifestyle on your own.

Many cancer survivors achieved self-discovery in some ways in the process of their survival. They obtained a new way of life for themselves by such enlightenment. This is not something special - anyone can experience it as long as they understand how the diseases are born.

From Abo Laboratory 7:
Reasons Why Doctors Rely on Medicine

In recent years, many people started to realize that modern medicine is not curing diseases at a satisfactory level. The reason for this is because the fundamental concept of modern medicine's treatment lies in the belief that the disease is bad and doctors prescribe medications to remove symptoms.

A German biochemist, Dr. Otto Warburg already discovered in the beginning of 20th century the fact that "cancer cell go through cell divisions by utilizing the energy produced by the glycolysis pathway which is not oxygen dependent".

Most of the diseases including cancer are caused as a result of an adaptive response of our bodies to the conditions of hypothermia and hypoxia.

We were close in identifying the causes of cancer in the time of Dr. Warburg, but for a long time, we didn't pay attention to the truth. This led to the drug dependent treatments which we can call "medicine that is unable to cure diseases".

I am positive that this reality will change as the true causes of diseases are revealed in this book.

Chapter 8: Important Things that Nutritional Science Has Forgotten About

Eating is Second in Priority

In the previous chapter, I mentioned that modern medicine are facing problems because it relies too heavily on prescribing medications for treating various diseases. In the chapters, I also mentioned that "dietary therapy" may be second in priority to focus on when treating diseases. Above all, what is most important is managing stress, which is also a main theme discussed in this book.

As I explained so far in the book, as long as we live, we will always experience stress in our lives. However, when the stress level in our daily lives increase and people fall into a situation where our bodies experience too much stress, thebodies respond to this emergency and try to adapt to the body environment. As a result, our bodies experience the state of hypoxia and hypothermia, the conditions where cancer cell divisions are encouraged.

Apparently, managing stress is very important to maintaining our health, because cancer can occur in our bodies when they try to adapt to the condition of hypoxia and hypothermia. This is why I say that changing what we eat is second in priority. What we should take care of first is stress.

We eat every day so contents of our daily diet are important, but our life is not only sustained and fueled by food.

There are some people who did not experience positive results of dietary therapy, or who could not continue with dietary therapy after trying it for a certain period of time. Probably, dietary therapy did not work for them not because there were issues with the methods, but because they might not have recognized in themselves that stress was a more important issue to take care of rather than taking care of the contents of their daily diet.

For example, **just constantly reminding ourselves that "I need to eat this because it is healthy for my body" can create stress. Also, being sensitive about foods by thinking that "this is bad for my body" or "that has carcinogens", etc. can impose stress on our bodies.**

Even though we eat healthy foods and take good supplements, if we do not deal with the stress that we have, these good things do not lead to an improvement in our bodies.

When I describe this in writing, many people think that these things are so simple and obvious. Although this might sound simple, it is human nature that once we focus on one perspective, it is hard to perceive things outside of the box. This tendency can also be seen in the individuals who are practicing dietary therapy.

It is good to keep in our minds that over-doing things can lead to losing a balance in our bodies even if what we are over-doing is something that is logical.

This applies not only to cancer, but other lifestyle related diseases like diabetes, hypertension and hyperlipidemia.

While keeping these things in mind, I would like to examine the root of the relationship between foods, health and stress in this chapter.

Sunlight is One of the Nutrients

Let's scrutinize the common consensus widely accepted in nutritional science.

In nutritional science, glucose (carbohydrate and glucide), protein, fat, minerals, vitamins are identified as the nutrients necessary for our bodies. Also, dietary fiber and phytochemical (i.e. polyphenol which is a plant pigment composition) are identified as nutrients. All of these cannot be synthesized within our bodies, so the only way for us to take in these nutrients are from eating foods.

From the perspective of nutritional science, as long as we ingest these nutrients in our bodies, our health is being maintained. But, is that really true?

We take in and digest nutrients from food through our intestines. The nutrients will be carried to all the cells by blood and used for the production of energy. Nutrients are necessary for both the glycolysis pathway and the mitochondrial pathway to produce energy.

However, nutrients are not all the resources needed for energy production. There are additional elements necessary for energy production in the mitochondrial pathway, for example, electromagnetic waves and low doses of radiation.

Many people are probably surprised when I mention that electromagnetic waves and radiation are necessary for energy production. Though these are harmful to our bodies, they do have some benefits too.

Electromagnetic waves exist in nature in different length of waves; gamma rays, X-ray, ultraviolet rays, visible rays, infrared rays and radio waves. Among these, the one that is necessary for our bodies is ultraviolet rays, and even more specifically, sunlight.

You might be surprised when I mention electromagnetic waves are necessary for our bodies. It might be easier to grasp this idea when I rephrase and explain that sunlight is important for our daily activities.

Taking in some sunlight, it activates the mitochondrial pathway and encourages energy productions. As a result, our bodies are warmed up comfortably. In contrast, when we stay home without going outside, we feel grim and do not feel energized. In this situation, the mitochondrial pathway is not stimulated for full production of energy. Even though a person takes in enough healthy nutrients, if there is no exposure to sunlight, the nutrients may not be able to convert enough energy for our bodies.

Now, I will explain the reasons why the sunlight activates mitochondria. I will do so by first examining the process of nutrients being converted to energy in mitochondria.

From page 38 in the section subtitled "Oxygen Produces Massive Energy", I mentioned this process. If I go into detail, it would be too complicated. Just keep in mind that as the nutrients are being broken down, hydrogen is being produced as an end product.

To produce energy for our daily activities, electric potential differences must be created between the inside and outside of the mitochondria's membrane by pulling apart the hydrogen molecule from nutrients via the electron transport chain. Hydrogen usually has a stable molecular structure, having consisted of one proton and one electron. In fact, sunlight, which is a type of electromagnetic wave, is doing this job of pulling apart hydrogen molecules.

You may now have a clearer idea of why eating nutritious foods is not enough to produce energy in the mitochondrial pathway.

It is important to re-

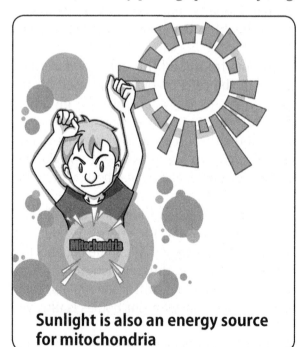

Sunlight is also an energy source for mitochondria

mind ourselves the importance of "being under sunlight" to stay healthy.

It is well known that chloroplasts in plants convert sunlight into energy. This applies to the mitochondrial pathway too. For many forms of life on the earth, sunlight is vital and necessary.

When we look at nutritional science from mitochondria as a starting point, then we can consider not only foods but also sunlight as nutrients.

Effects of Low Dose Radiation Contained in Vegetables

Let me further explain the relationship between sunlight rays and health.

I mentioned earlier that we feel great as we take a walk outside in the sun, because mitochondria are being activated by sunlight. This correlates with the idea that I have explained repeatedly in this book that "mitochondria become activated in warm temperatures".

Moderation is also important as we have a proverb that says "too much is as bad as too little". There is a limit in how much we should warm our bodies as too much heat will damage cells which can trigger apoptosis (programmed death of cells).

When we sunbathe too much, we may get sunstroke or heatstroke. This situation symbolizes the cry of the mitochondria telling us "we cannot take much more heat". When we do not listen to the warning and continue to warm our bodies, then cells go into apoptosis and can end our lives suddenly.

Dizziness caused by taking a long hot bath is also caused by warming up the mitochondria too much. I will explain in details about this case later on.

To stimulate mitochondria, the balance in temperature as well as the frequency and length of being in the moderate temperature is important as either too much warming or too much cooling can affect the mitochondria negatively.

Now, let's take a look at rays from radiation.

No one probably likes the image of "exposure to radiation". However, radiation rays exist in nature, and we all are exposed to them as in a similar way as we are exposed to electromagnetic rays in our daily lives.

Of course, the balance is important in this case too. When we are exposed to too much radiation, our bodies may not function properly. As a doctor, I am hesitant to recommend radiation therapy, because the dose of radiation patients will be exposed to during therapy is high. High doses of radiation may alter cells and these cells may also have a negative effect on surrounding cells.

More specifically, radiation may damage the cell membrane and the acidified contents inside of the exploded cells can come into contact with the normal cells around them and affect them negatively. Such damage is more severe than the damage caused by chemotherapy, and it will take a long time before complete recovery.

However, the radiation that exists in nature is much lower in dosage than that of radiation therapy. It gives a good stimulus for our bodies. Surprisingly, a low dose of radiation is contained in vegetables and fruits.

What is Included in Vegetables but Not in Supplements?

This low dose of radiation contained in vegetables and fruits are called kalium-40 (potassium-40).

Kalium-40 is one of the minerals which have existed since the earth was born. Kalium-40 has one extra neutron than regular kalium, so it tries to stabilize itself by releasing a very low level of radiation to become a proton.

However, its natural abundance is only 0.012%, and its half-life is 1.26 billion years. Its leap does not even reach 1mm, so just by touching vegetables and fruits do not result in an exposure to radiation.

When this dose of radiation is being taken inside of our bodies and carried to the cells, the leap is a good distance. This distance allows the low doses of radiation which is contained in the kalium-40 to come into contact with mitochondria within the cells. During this process, hydrogen is pulled apart from the nutrients.

As I explained so far, nutrients contained in food are being broken down in various stages when they are carried inside of cells. At the end of these complex processes, hydrogen is taken out in the electron transport chain within the mitochondria.

Kalium- 40 is a necessary element in the process of pulling hydrogen out of nutrients, as important as the energy from sunlight.

In short, **intake of vegetables and fruits are important not only because we can take in nutrients such as glucose, vitamins and minerals, but also we can take in kalium-40, a low dosage of radiation in our bodies.**

In the previous chapter, I explained when there is more natrium in the outer cell and more kalium in the inside of the cell, the mineral within the cells in our bodies is balanced. The reasons why our cells wanted to absorb kalium was not clearly understood until recently.

However, when we understand the characteristics of kalium, we then understand that the reason was that the mitochondria required our cells to take in radiation.

When we eat fresh vegetables and fruits, we feel like being re-born. This is because our bodies can rebound from tiredness with the supply of kalium- 40. Our bodies can then activate the energy production in mitochondria.

To explain this mechanism in detail, animals ingest kalium by eating plants. Plants absorb kalium from soil to grow. Three main elements in fertilizer are nitrogen, phosphoric acid and kalium.

Also, kalium-40 changes to calcium after breaking down by releasing radiation. A Periodic Table of Elements indicates that the next element to kalium is calcium. Our bodies can produce calcium from kalium-40 which releases radiation. This means, as long as we eat enough vegetables, we will have enough intake of calcium then. You may not need to force yourself to drink milk just because you are concerned about your calcium intake.

Vitamins and minerals contained in the vegetables and fruits are important nutrients for mitochondria, but that is not all. Additions of low doses of radiation and electromagnetic waves also stimulate energy production in the powerhouse of the mitochondrial pathways.

By taking supplements and vitamin tablets, you are not taking in radiation that is necessary for mitochondria to be activated. Eating fresh vegetables and fruits cultivated from nature can provide nutrients and radiation necessary for activating the mitochondria.

Why Are There Healthy People Among Hyper-Light-Eaters?

Actually, there is another element that I should mention, other than the radiation and electromagnetic waves. That is oxygen.

Oxygen is inhaled into our bodies by breathing and taken into the blood through the bronchi in the lungs. Oxygen is carried to cells all over our bodies through the blood just like nutrients.

I explained that the ancestor of mitochondria was aerobic bacteria which could convert oxygen into energy. So, mitochondria have characteristics that are activated in aerobic exercises, which means, when our bodies are lacking oxygen, then energy productions in our bodies are also stalled. As a result of lacking oxygen, we may feel that we do not have enough energy.

To explain this in relationship with the mechanism of energy productions, hydrogen which is pulled apart inside of mitochondria will be combined with oxygen to turn them into water. Energy is produced in this process.

Low doses of radiation, electromagnetic waves, oxygen···understanding the importance of these factors may now give you an idea that the conventional understanding of nutritional science may not explain the entirety of health. In other words, there is always the reality of facts that cannot be explained by conventional understanding or common sense.

For example, it is widely understood that each adult requires about 1200 - 1500 kilo calories for basal metabolism each day. If you exercise, more calories are needed. However, there are a few people who are living healthy lives every day without eating foods that match this basal metabolism, just like hermits.

For instance, astonishingly, Ms. Michiyo Mori who lives in Osaka, Japan, has been drinking only one glass of green vegetable juice (80 kilo calories) per day for the last 15 years.

80 kilo calories equals to one glass of soy milk. A regular person like us will not even last several days. From the nutritional science point of view, it is improbable and many exclaim that this is "unthinkable" and "impossible".

Foods are not all nutrients for our bodies

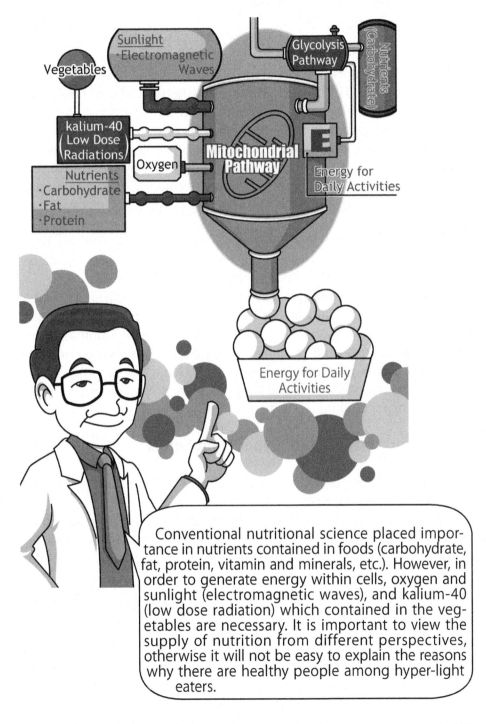

Conventional nutritional science placed importance in nutrients contained in foods (carbohydrate, fat, protein, vitamin and minerals, etc.). However, in order to generate energy within cells, oxygen and sunlight (electromagnetic waves), and kalium-40 (low dose radiation) which contained in the vegetables are necessary. It is important to view the supply of nutrition from different perspectives, otherwise it will not be easy to explain the reasons why there are healthy people among hyper-light eaters.

In reality, she is very healthy and handles her acupuncture practice every day as well. Her diet is amazingly little, but she is not super skinny, but rather of medium build.

Also, I have co-authored a book called "A person who lives, barely eating" with Mr. Toshihiko Shibata. Every day, he has eaten food totaling about 500 kilo calories, consisting of brown rice and vegetables for a period of one year. His body changed for the better and now he lives his life happily, physically and mentally improved.

Before he started to challenge this hyper-low calorie diet, he was warned by a nutritional science professional that "If you continue such diets, you will lose your weight dramatically and may die". During the diet, he had a check up with his doctor, but his medical data was normal. Not only did he believe himself to be healthy, but it is proven by medical data as well.

The cases of these two individuals may be at an extreme, but there are people who live healthy by eating little which might be considered reckless from the perspective of nutritional science.

I will go over the reasons why in detail later on, but in short, "eating is not all". **As long as we have certain conditions in our bodies, humans can adapt to the daily habit of "barely eating". Rather, humans have historically experienced periods of hunger, so eating small portions suit the human's physiologies better.** Nutritional science only look at nutrients from foods, and because of this view, it hinders providing the effective tips for leading a true healthy life.

A Look Inside Intestines of Hyper-Light-Eaters

Many professionals were curious about Ms. Mori's uncommon hyper-light diet and many researched on her.

The most important one is the research done on the conditions of her intestinal bacteria. When we checked on her feces, there were higher than normal numbers of bacteria that broke down the cellulose (fiber) of plants were found.

Our intestine cannot digest fibers contained in foods usually, so fibers come out of our bodies as feces. However, bacteria in Ms. Mori's intestines break down fibers and produce amino acid.

When amino acid is carried to cells, it is synthesized into protein, a nutrient. This was the reasons why she can continue to live by drinking a glass of green vegetable juice a day, and her body can build muscles by eating only vegetables.

This may sounds a little mysterious, but herbivores such as cows and horse can maintain such masculine bodies. It can be explained by their eating habits - eating bacteria with dry grass and consequently increasing the numbers of bacteria in their intestines.

In a way, Ms. Mori's intestine is the same as that of herbivores.

Also, there is another very interesting research data reported about Ms. Mori in the field of immunology, which is the field I specialize in. It was confirmed that when Ms. Mori's blood concentration level of Interferon-alpha was measured, it was 4 times higher than that of regular adults. Interferon-alpha is a kind of immunomodulating agent in our blood and is known for suppressing the division of cancer cells. We can assume that Mr. Mori's immunity potential is very high.

In chapter 4, I have mentioned that the macrophages which are one of defensive cells process nutrients in addition to eating virus and bacteria.

When we overeat, macrophages need to process nutrients and as a result, they expand so much which slows down the biological defense.

We imagine that we are healthier when we take a lot of nutrients into our bodies. But in reality, when we eat less, the immunity is strengthened more. As a result, we can build healthy bodies.

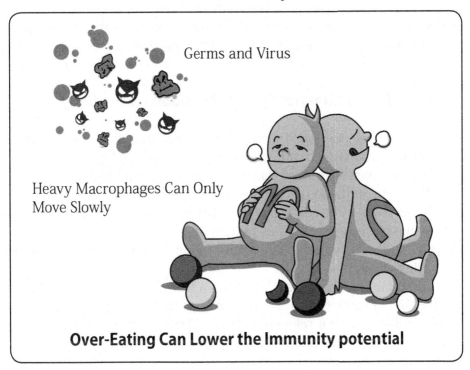

Germs and Virus

Heavy Macrophages Can Only Move Slowly

Over-Eating Can Lower the Immunity potential

In nutritional science, calculation of calories is often mentioned. This method digitizes the energy burned per food.

By using this method, nutritional science calculate the calories required for each day. As an example, 1 gram of glucose (carbohydrate, glucide) and protein equals to 4 kilo calories and 1 gram of fat as 9 kilo calories, etc. However, our bodies do not produce energy by burning the foods.

The main source of energy is glucose. When glucose is broken down in the glycolysis pathway, it is broken down to pyruvic acid and lactic acid. Energy produced in this process is very little. Pyruvic acid is then carried to mitochondria and massive energy is produced there by also adding electromagnetic waves and radiation.

As I mentioned in this chapter, the last stage of energy production in our bodies goes through the process: "hydrogen + oxygen = water". Energy is obtained in different forms in the last stage of energy production, rather than processing and burning the foods. Also, there are other elements added along the process. This is a reason why there is a gap between understanding what nutritional science offers and health in reality.

There is a real person in India who has been living only by drinking water. This is neither a miracle nor a mysterious thing. This person's body produces enough energy while not relying on foods. And, this can be explained in some degree from a physiological perspective.

Reasons Why Radium Hot Springs Are Good for the Body

So far, I have identified some of the issues that nutritional science has. Actually, radiation that I explained previously can be taken into our bodies in another way, other than from vegetables and fruits.

That is by utilizing the radium contained in soil and rocks.

In the crust of the earth, it is said that more than 100 kinds of radioactive substances exist, such as radium and kalium-40. In Japan where most of the land is volcanic landforms, radium is often contained in the hot spring water.

To explain in more detail, radium is a substance that is a variable of radioactive substance such as uranium and thorium. Radium is an unstable substance and it releases radiation when broken down and turns into gas such as radon and thoron.

Radium hot springs gushed forth while passing through near the mineral rocks such as uranium and thorium in the deep underground. So, when we are taking a bath and inhaling the steam of radium hot springs, we can take in low doses of radiation all over our bodies.

Taking a bath in hot springs is healthy for our bodies. It encourages better blood flow in our bodies and relaxation. Positive effects of taking hot spring baths are proven by the fact that the mitochondria prefer the warmer environment.

In radium hot springs, in addition to keeping our bodies warm, low doses of radiation further encourage energy production by mitochondria.

Between 1970s and 1980s, the American biochemist, Dr. Thomas Luckey researched on how the low dose of radiation positively affects human bodies.

He named the positive health effect of the low doses of radiations as hormesis, which means "radiation that has similar effects as hormones". He raised a question to the conventional understanding of radiation that it is toxic to human bodies even in low level exposure.

At his time, the public image toward radiation was even more negative than that of now, so his research was not spotlighted then. However, after his time, the research lived on and in recent years, the positive effects of low dosages of radiation were slowly confirmed by various researches.

I, myself, have been investigating hormesis with mice. When we irradiate one forty fifth of a lethal dose of radiation on a mouse for a certain period, I could confirm that the immune strength of the mouse increased slowly but steadily.

In reality, there are many people who were cured of cancer by taking hot spring baths for a period of time as treatment at the Tamagawa Hot Springs in Akita Prefecture as well as Misasa Hot Springs in Tottori Prefecture in Japan where they are known for radium hot springs. Beitou hot spring in Taiwan and hot spring in Bad Gastein in Austria are also well-known radium hot springs. People also report cases of various diseases including cancers being cured by taking a bath in radium hot springs for a period of time in these locations, too.

The reasons why radium hot springs have a positive effect on curing cancers is that taking a bath there create a synergistic effect of hyperthermia and hormesis, and that encourages the energy production by the mitochondria.

When mitochondria are activated, then divisions of the cancer cells which get divided via the glycolysis pathway are discouraged, leading to the spontaneous remission of cancer cells.

There was an epidemiological study done in the area of Misasa Hot Springs. It is confirmed that the people who live in the neighborhood of Misasa Hot Springs only have a half of the death rate from cancer compared to the national average in Japan.

After working hard for many years, people may fall into the body environment where hypothermia and hypoxia became the norm. If these people can take getting a cancer as an opportunity to truly rest their bodies, to re-examine how they lived so far, and to come up with how they want to live their future lives while relaxing in a natural hot spring, that would be a wonderful thing.

As I explained in this book so far, cancers can be spontaneously cured **if we can prepare our bodies to be under certain conditions where it is hard for cancer cells to survive.**

Did the Sen'nin, Immortal Hermits of the Mountain, have Hypothermia?

Let's go back to talk about nutritional science again. I have examined the mechanism of how light eaters are living healthy. However, it does not mean that we all cannot become healthy just because we do not imitate the daily diet of "not eating much".

Humans have lived through a long period of hunger in history. Because of this, whenever humans get food to eat, then we tend to eat a lot, letting our bodies fall into the glycolysis pathway dominant environment.

In order for us to fully utilize the ineffective energy from the glycolysis pathway, our bodies require constant intake of nutrients (mainly glucose). As a result, if a period of time without glucose last too long, our bodies get hungry easily and we feel a strong craving for food. This is the reason why we have psychological difficulties in cutting down food intake or trying not to eat a meal.

If we ignore these desires for foods, and force ourselves into light eating or fasting, then it can cause low blood glucose levels which can cause sickness to our bodies.

However, if you tend to stuff yourselves with food regularly or have lifestyle related diseases now, then you should start eating less or practice eating until 80% full, while understanding the mechanism of human bodies as I explained in this book. You should do this at your own pace, taking it step by step.

To distance ourselves from eating enough meals a day and to distance ourselves from the glycolysis pathway takes time getting used to. For Ms. Mori to be able to live her daily life by only drinking a glass of green vegetable juice a day, it took her several years to become accustomed to that lifestyle. She also tried various eating habits and methods in the course of those years.

If you start practicing fasting or eating light, then please keep in mind that there will be the glycolysis pathway resisting the new eating habit. Again, do this at your own pace and take your time to train your bodies.

After all, if you do not have big diseases such as cancer, then you do not need to practice eating light. Especially if you are young, then your bodies produce energy via the glycolysis pathway dominantly. So, it is more natural that you eat what you want to eat and engage in activities energetically.

As I explained in Chapter 4, as we age, human bodies shift toward dominant energy production by the mitochondrial pathway naturally. This means that we will have more endurance as time goes on. As we get older, we eat less food too, due to this shift in energy production in our bodies.

At the end of this spectrum are hermits. We can consider people who can live while eating hyper-light as individuals who reached a step closer to being hermits by training themselves.

In general, healthy people have higher basal body temperature (around 36.5° C/97.7° F) and have masculine bodies. However, people who are hyper-light eaters have lower basal body temperature (around 36° C/96.8° F) and are not so masculine. These are exceptional people who obtained the body which can use energy very efficiently by utilizing the energy production via mitochondrial pathway. Their bodies can certainly deal with hunger.

What Does the Energy Convert to When Carbohydrate (Sugar, Glucose) Intake is Reduced?

When we view fasting and eating light as a shift from the energy production via the glycolysis pathway to the mitochondrial pathway, we can consider that is also one way of living our lives naturally. Besides eating light, there is also another way to shift utilizing energy from the glycolysis pathway to the mitochondrial pathway.

That would be limiting the glucose intake, which has been spotlighted in the field of medicine recently.

By limiting the glucose intake, it means literally to limit the intake of glucose (carbohydrate such as rice, bread, noodles, sugar, and potato products, etc.) It is commonly used as a treatment option for treating diabetes. Because the glycolysis pathway produces its energy from glucose, so when we do not supply it with glucose, then the glycolysis pathway naturally shrinks.

Fasting shrinks the glycolysis pathway by not eating foods at all. By limiting the glucose intake, it targets the main energy fuel to the glycolysis pathway. By limiting the main fuel to the glycolysis pathway, it can encourage the production of energy via the mitochondrial pathway.

It may seem like a simple method, but if you have some knowledge of nutritional science, then you may have a question; "By limiting the glucose intake, how can people produce enough energy for daily activities?"

In fact, it is true that the mitochondrial pathway is fueled by the nutrients broken down by the glycolysis pathway. So, it is logical to think that when we limit the glucose intake, then it will affect the efficiency of the energy production in the mitochondrial pathway. Especially since we have understood that the brain can only be fueled by glucose, and it is true that the lack of glucose intake can cause a lack of focus.

When people fast, they do not completely cut off the glucose intake. This is to prevent the body from falling into extreme hypoglycemia.

This understanding of the mechanism in our bodies is correct. However, recent studies start to reveal that our bodies react differently when we limit the glucose intake.

Our bodies are mainly maintained by three major nutrients, glucose, protein and fat.

Among these three, glucose can be converted to energy the fastest. But when our bodies lack glucose, then protein and after that fat will be used for producing the energy.

To explain this in a bit more in detail, protein is converted to amino acid and fat is converted to a fatty acid before our body cells can absorb them. Both of them are broken down in mitochondria to fuel the energy productions.

Amino acid and fatty acid do not go through the glycolysis pathway so they may not lead to instantaneous force productions. However, because of this mechanism, lack of glucose intake may not affect the more dominant energy production house, the mitochondrial pathway, because protein and fat can fuel the mitochondria when our bodies lack glucose.

Among these fuels, the most spotlighted one in recent years is fat.

Fat contained in foods will be broken down into fatty acid first. When fatty acid is being carried to the liver, it changes to a substance called ketone. This ketone will then be carried to cells in our bodies and become fuel to the energy production house in the mitochondria.

The ketone which is converted from fat can obviously be used by the brain as energy too. Common knowledge about how brains need glucose is actually not an absolute idea.

Why Does the Body Temperature Rise When Carbohydrate Intake is Reduced?

The increase of the ketone has been reported among serious diabetic patients whose pancreases have difficulties secreting insulin and are unable to utilize the glucose.

This state is called ketosis and is a condition which is viewed as critical in the conventional treatment field of diabetes. However, when people successfully adapted to limiting the glucose intake, even if they have the condition of ketosis, they do not suffer from health concerns. Rather, they can live their lives perfectly fine, better than regular people.

Moreover, in these cases, glucose intake is strictly limited, so that the blood glucose level can be stabilized. Because of this, patients can no longer need to depend upon the conventional medications such as hypoglycemic agents and insulin injections, even if they are having ketosis which has been considered as a critical condition traditionally by the field of medicine.

You might be puzzled by now, but in a different view, this makes sense. By limiting the glucose intake, this removes the direct cause of increase in the blood glucose level and allows the pancreas functions to rest. It is logical that the conditions move toward remission.

In contrast, conventional treatments of diabetes lack the concept of limiting the glucose intake. Even though limiting the intake of daily calories, patients will continue to take in some level of glucose. In this treatment however, patients may continue to rely on the glycolysis pathway. This may not lead to the improvement of the diabetic conditions, but may result in worsening conditions.

In Japan, the diabetes treatment by limiting the glucose intake has been gradually spreading. A doctor who is in the center of this movement is Dr. Toyoaki Kamaike in the Ehime Prefecture.

Many people who heard this treatment method are naturally surprised. Doctors who use this method will instruct patients to strictly limit the glucose intake. So, there is no carbohydrate intake in the patients' diet, cutting rice and breads. Also, patients will not eat any sweets such as cakes.

On the other hand, intake of proteins such as meats increases. Doctors usually suggest patients to eat more vegetables, too, which prevent negative effect to the intestines by providing fibers which are lacking if people only eat proteins.

When we compare this with the conventional treatment of diabetes, this method is more logical. As a reader of this book, you might also realize that this method also meet the fundamental needs of human health.

As I mentioned, when we think about health, "issues of stress need to be taken care of before thinking about daily diets".

Fundamentally, diabetes is also caused by stress. Actually, the body environment of hyperglycemia is the condition resulting from our bodies trying to respond to the emergency caused by stress. So, diabetes is a condition where bodies are responding to the stress.

When glucose is limited, then the energy productions via the glycolysis pathway become less dominant. Then, mitochondria become dominant in producing energy. As a result, bodies can escape from the hypothermia and hypoxia as the conditions of diabetes itself also improves slowly. When our bodies experience this positive change, then we naturally start feeling relaxed and are stabilized emotionally. Going through this change allows us to escape from the stressful lifestyle as well.

In my opinion, improvements of hyperglycemia by implementing a change in daily diets are just a surface of how our bodies react. It is not absolute. When this method fits particular patients' lifestyle in positive ways and they are also successful in taking care of their stress, this method becomes effective in allowing patients to escape from hyperglycemia. When choosing treatment options, it is also necessary to determine the compatibility with our own lifestyles, too.

Should You Force Yourself to Be a Light-Eater?

I would like to mention again that if we do not consciously be attentive about how stress plays a role in maintaining our health, people who practice fasting or eating light can only focus on daily food intake.

When we limit what we eat every day, it means to limit our desires by thinking "I want to eat this, but I cannot eat this". This can cause stress. So, some people may not be fit to limit what they eat every day or eat lightly.

People who succeed in dietary therapy are ones who are pulled into the method by an opportunity and happened to be able to adapt to the methods. There are so many people who failed in dietary therapy because the success rate is rather opportunistic. This may explain the reason why this method is not widely spread out.

As I mentioned repeatedly in this book, humans live by balancing the energy production utilizing both the glycolysis pathway and the mitochondrial pathway. Both instantaneous force and endurance are necessary for us to survive.

When people become sick because they rely on the energy production via the glycolysis pathway, then they need to weaken the dependency to the glycolysis pathway to obtain a healthy life. As one of the methods to achieve that goal, it can be effective to implement some sort of dietary regulations. However, as I explained, if you are in the age group between 20s and 50s then it is not natural to completely cut off the energy production via the glycolysis pathway.

It is a personal choice to decide whether you want to start living like hermits early in your life. That is up to you. But, if you consider living like hermits at an earlier age is a norm, then it may result in losing balance in your bodies.

What is most important is how you can deal with your stress. In that bigger goal, the daily diet is included as an optional solution.

We need to understand the health conditions such as hyperglycemia and hypertension are our bodies' physiological adaptive responses informing us about the imbalance in our current lifestyles. It is not all about the imbalance in what we eat every day.

If a person has been diligently following the dietary therapy method by believing what she or he eats changes health conditions, that person might have forgotten about the issues relating to stress and how the lifestyle of the person has been. People who succeed in dietary therapy may suggest to people who are struggling with sickness that they should "change your daily diets". It is most likely suggested with good intentions. However, we also need to understand that the dietary therapy is not all and to note that some cases reported that dietary therapies are not effective.

For people who have been implementing dietary therapy and it has been going well, than please continue with that. However, if you are practicing the dietary therapy for a while and do not feel any positive change, then you might need to realize how important it is to first deal with stress.

You may realize that you have been tolerating something that you did not want to do. By realizing that, then you will naturally be able to start focusing and reassessing how you want to live your life. Once you can do this, then your conditions of hyperglycemia will probably improve, even though you do not implement strict dietary restrictions for everyday foods.

Diabetes Come from the Lifestyle

I would like to analyze at the end about the mechanism of having diabetes, as I spent time talking about limiting the glucose intake in this chapter.

In general, diabetes gets worse when insulin which lowers the blood glucose level is no longer secreted. So, usually doctors prescribe hypoglycemic drugs to patients to help lower the secretion of insulin, to control the blood glucose level.

Patients' bodies need to process a lot of glucose, so in a way, patients' bodies are secreting more insulin than healthy persons.

In modern medicine, we call "insulin resistance" when hyperglycemia is not improving even though there seems to be enough production of insulin. By this, doctors conclude that this occurs because insulin itself lost its effectiveness. However, there is a contradiction in this understanding.

By coming up with a new vague concept to explain the condition, while trying to somehow connect the dots, does not allow us to see the fundamental truth about diabetes.

As I mentioned earlier, diabetes can be caused by stress. Stress can cause hypoxia and hypothermia, and if we do not look at this issue, then we may not be able to see the fundamental truth of the cause of diabetes.

In fact, the true cause of the lack of improvement on hyperglycemia even though there is enough secretion of insulin is the body environment where bodies are not utilizing enough glucose from our blood.

Low use of glucose in the blood means that the energy productions in the cells are not being processed efficiently.

It means that there is a surplus of glucose because mitochondria are not working effectively.

Then, the question is; why are the mitochondria not working effectively? We can conclude that it is due to the overuse of the glycolysis pathway. However, when we look at it from the physiological view, mitochondria do not work effectively because our bodies are at the state of hypoxia and hypothermia.

In short, **continuous state of hypoxia and hypothermia lead to the low use of glucose in the blood.**

The issue in particular is hypothermia. To prove this, when we take the temperature of diabetic patients, all of them have hypothermia without exception. As a result, many patients may have swollen legs due to the lack of energy and also have weakened kidneys.

When we follow this lead, then we can reveal the effective ways to cure diabetes.

First of all the fundamental key is to keep our bodies warm, for example, by taking a bath and to change the lifestyles if we overwork. In relation to foods, when people overwork, they tend to overeat as well. When we overeat, then we tend to take in too much glucose. This can happened because our bodies tried to take in more nutrients when the utilization rate of glucose is low and our bodies lack energy. As a result, the glycolysis pathway becomes dominant in energy production.

The fundamental cause is due to stress that people expose themselves to every day. Dietary therapy is one option to deal with the condition, but what is most important is to deal with the stress. This applies not only to diabetes, but also to other lifestyle related diseases.

When we realize what the nutritional science did not pick up, then the issue of stress and individuals' lifestyles becomes clear as a cause for diabetes.

From Abo Laboratory 8: Is Nutritional Science Useless?

The main reason why we eat food every day is to supply nutrients to cells and produce energy in the mitochondria. However, the fuel for energy production is not only food.

As I explained in this chapter, oxygen, sunlight and radiations contained in vegetables are all important "nutrients" that fuel the mitochondria.

Unfortunately, in nutritional science textbooks, there is no mention of these additional nutrients other than food. This caused many people to believe that the importance lies with having "well-balanced foods".

However, this understanding missed some important tips on living our lives in a healthy way.

It is a theme for the 21st Century to establish a "new nutritional science" which should be more useful to our health, and to establish a new medical practice which is true to the law of living beings.

Chapter 9: Eight Rules for Staying Away
from Cancer

The Best Prescriptions Are Achieved by Improving Your Lifestyle

I believe that what I have revealed in my book is the ultimate answer to a question which has been asked by many people: "Why do people get sick?" My response is obviously clear. I have formulated my answer from the secrets of the human souls and bodies, so I am confident that it is the solution.

In this last chapter, I would like to think about things we should keep in mind every day in order to stay away from cancer, which is one of the most deadly diseases around the world.

When we ask ourselves the question of "why do people get cancer?", I believe it will lead us to re-examine how we live every day. We are accustomed to going to a hospital when we get sick so that doctors can cure the sickness. Obviously, this is far from being conscious about our lifestyles each day.

Some medical treatments are necessary and effective, but modern medicine considers that disease is caused by failure in our bodies. The conventional medicine's approach to disease-which is to remove the affected areas and illness-is far from following the path of true health. As I mentioned, many illnesses can be caused by an imbalance in our own lifestyles. To obtain true health, we need to first change our perception in this regard.

In fact, we can also say that not focusing on our everyday lifestyles might have caused an increase in the numbers of cancer patients.

In the areas of western medicine, eastern medicine and alternative medicine, various treatment options for cancer patients have been introduced. What is the most important to note in developing a cure for cancer is, **not "how to cure cancer", but to understand the "mechanism of getting cancer" and the importance of maintaining a balance in our lifestyles. It may sound simple, but this can be a powerful prescription to treat cancer.**

What treatment options should we use? What types of foods and exercises should we eat or do? By understanding the importance of maintaining a balance in our lifestyles, answers to these questions become clearer and more meaningful to us. Reacting to the symptoms of cancer and focusing upon ways to remove or control the symptoms can distant us from seeing the truth: "cancer is a common disease", which I mentioned in my book repeatedly.

Cancer is an adaptive response to hypothermia and hypoxia. It is a wonderful wisdom that our bodies have been equipped with.

Then, we should utilize this wisdom instead of trying to remove or stop it.

This applies to many diseases. Many people become either happy or worried about their bodies when they see the results on medical examination reports from annual checkups. However, it is essential for us to view these checkup results with an understanding that many medical conditions such as hyperglycemia and hypertension (high blood pressure) are an adaptive response of our bodies. When we all do so, then our reactions while viewing the results will change.

Importance of Knowing What to Prioritize

What I said so far in this chapter is basically what I explained in detail in my book. As you can see, my explanations do not match the conventional common sense that modern medicine has taught us so far. So, I understand if readers get astonished by my explanation, especially those who have been told that contracting diseases are very scary things. I also understand if they feel a little confused.

Also, I would imagine readers would probably like to learn more practical details in terms of how to maintain balance in their lifestyles.

Therefore, as a conclusion of this book, I would like to introduce "eight rules for staying away from cancer".

Please be conscious about keeping a balance in how you live every day and if you notice an unbalancing factor in your lifestyle when referring to the following eight rules, then please try to improve that at your own pace. If there is a time when you feel uncertain about how you can adjust the situation, please read over my book again. You will probably be able to encounter and pick up a new tip every time you open the book.

So here they are. Eight rules for staying away from cancer are the following:

1. Be Aware of Physical and Mental Stress
2. Change the Lifestyle of Being Too Diligent
3. Find Ways to Take a Break and Relax
4. Be Creative about Not Cooling Down Your Body
5. Replace Excessive Drinking and Eating with Light Eating
6. Integrate Aerobic Exercise in Your Lifestyle
7. Cherish Good Laughs and Show Your Gratitude
8. Have a Purpose in Life, Find Joy in Your Lifetime and Set Goals

All these rules are essentially what I mentioned in this book. Please note though, these items are numbered by priority. So, the lower numbered items are the first ones you should be conscious of. Instead of trying to keep all eight rules at once, please begin by incorporating the lower numbered items one by one, 1, 2, 3 then 4···

Especially 1, 2 and 3 are the core foundation of being able to stay away from developing the conditions of hypothermia and hypoxia which can cause cancer.

People who are already incorporating dietary therapy or alternative medicine might already be practicing 4-6, but they might have forgotten or are not including items 1-3.

By diligently trying not to cool down the body, or being very strict about improving their eating habits or exercising, our bodies can fall under stress. Although they follow these more visible rules diligently, people may hardly think about their unbalanced lifestyle or worries which are not so visible to us. Stress caused by these factors can lead to hypothermia and hypoxia, which ironically can cause cancer. So, being aware and conscious about stress is most important.

If you are now wondering "Why are my conditions or medical symptoms not improving even though I followed all the suggestions from doctors?" then, you need to realize the stress that you are imposing on yourself by strictly following these suggestions. When you realize that, then you will probably be able to move a step forward toward a cancer-free life.

It is more important to discover what kinds of tendency or imbalance you have in your lifestyles rather than trying to figure out how you will not have any cancer in your body. When you discover that, then naturally, you will be able to create a daily diet and exercise plan that suit yourself.

In regards to the last two items, 7 and 8, you can start incorporating these after you feel confident that you are now keeping the rules 1-6. By then, you will have enough space mentally and physically to focus on these broader goals. If you try to incorporate these two rules from the beginning, you may get stressed out and will not be able to maintain these goals. So, please do this step by step at your own pace, and it is fine to give yourself some time.

Now, I will try to explain each item in more detail.

Be Aware of Physical and Mental Stress

We are so busy every day and tend not to be attentive about how much stress or worries that our bodies and souls are withstanding each day. As we push ourselves while not dealing with the stress or worries accumulating daily, various symptoms occur in our bodies.

The most obvious one is the color of our face.

People also may start having headaches, shoulder pains, back pains, stomach pain, constipation, insomnia and menstrual pain due to the imbalance in the Autonomic Nervous System (ANS).

Stomatitis and skin issues such as dry skin are also signs of stress. By pausing and noticing these signs of stress, you are having conversations with your soul and heart. This process is very important.

When you have pain, it is essential to understand the cause of such pain, rather than reacting to the pain and trying to focus on removing the symptoms.

When you think about the cause, you may realize that it exists near you. You may find it in the interpersonal relationships that you have been worrying about. Or, you may find it in the career or personal goals that you feel that you have not fully achieved.

There are different ways to notice these signs. You may talk to someone about your stress. You may want to write them down. Even if a lot of things may not always offer you quick solutions, identifying them sometimes help to reduce the stress level and calm overwhelming feelings down.

Please make time and give yourself space to relax where you can converse with yourself.

Change the Lifestyle of Being Too Diligent

When you are able to make time and space to reflect upon your stress or worries, then the next step is to try to change your lifestyle of being too serious and diligent.

Many cancer patients are diligent people who take their responsibilities too seriously. These types of people tend to juggle multiple responsibilities on their own shoulders, from responsibilities at work and chores at home. Also, these people tend to carry and hold on to anger and complaints. They may furrow their brows all the time.

In the society, outcomes of their lifestyles may be praised, but if they are always feeling the pressure to be diligent and serious, then the pressure may lead them to sickness. Please reflect upon your lifestyle by asking the following questions: "Do you tend to work overtime all the time?"; "Is the effort absolutely necessary?"; "Can some of these assignments be delegated to someone else?" Please reflect on these things regularly.

Our bodies sustain activities in daily lives by keeping an intricate balance of complex functions such as the glycolysis pathway, the mitochondrial pathway, the SNS and PNS, granulocytes and leukocytes. It is unnecessary to let our bodies respond to emergency situations all the time, while sustaining our stressful lives by turning our body cells into cancer cells so we can survive the situation.

It is critical to relax and operate at minimum at times. By doing so, you may be surprised at how enjoyable your life is and may find yourself being more productive at your work.

Find Ways to Take a Break and Relax

The third step is to find ways to take a break and relax.

Allocating time to relax and have a break is also essential in addition to not to being too diligent or serious at work and doing house chores. 1 and 2 are probably easy to understand, but to implement them fully in real life is probably difficult. So, try to balance between on and off times well. When you need to put 100% into something important, try hard. But, after doing so, give yourself a break and do something fun and relax, something that you can gain a positive energy from. Please be mindful about utilizing the on and off switch of your seriousness and diligence wisely.

To change from your constant serious face, you may need to find a new hobby that you can enjoy when you are free. You should have another face separate from working or doing chores at home.

If you are the kind of person who works all the time, start from making some time to spend with your family. That step forward can make a big difference.

If you are the kind of person who has naturally been practicing 1-3, then you probably live a healthy life where you have a good balance in your body and soul.

Even though you have already been practicing a balanced lifestyle or have been conscious about it, there will always be times when the balance collapses. When that happens, what is important is to think about your physical health. So, being attentive about daily diets and exercising, or implementing other methods to achieve physical health are very important.

But, the question is where to begin.

Be Creative about Not Cooling Down Your Body

The first thing I would like to recommend is "not cooling down your body". It is the same thing as "keeping your body warm" or "maintaining a higher body temperature", but this is a big secret to maintaining our physical health.

The best indication of this is the basal body temperature (BBT). Around 36.5 ° C (97.7° F) is a barometer of health. As you stay up late at night or have a hangover, your BBT decrease by 0.3 ° C (≒0.5° F). When you are in such conditions, do not push yourself and leave work early. Take a long bath and make sure to have enough sleep at night. By doing so, the BBT will go back to the normal range.

Women are especially dependent on the mitochondrial pathway for energy production, so women's bodies can be more sensitive to a lower body temperature. Please be attentive about not drinking too many cold drinks, or wearing too little clothing. It might be a good idea to go to the sauna, hot spring, or stone baths. Of course, men should also be attentive about keeping their bodies warm. It is good to build muscles by appropriately utilizing the energy produced in the glycolysis pathway to increase metabolism and muscle. Masculine people have better metabolism, so as a result, they have warmer bodies.

Please note the difference between female and male bodies, and utilize the differences to come up with your own ways to keep your body warm.

Replace Excessive Drinking and Eating with Light Eating

To stay away from hypothermia and hypoxia, it is important to be conscious about what and how we eat every day. The foundation of a good daily diet is to eat vegetables that are rich in kalium-40 (potassoim-40) which can activate mitochondria in our cells every day.

Incorporate millets and brown rice that are rich in minerals, vitamins and fibers as a main dish. These foods also maintain intestinal functions. It is also important to eat fish, beans, seaweed and mushrooms, so be creative in incorporating these ingredients into your daily cooking.

When you eat vegetables, eat more varieties such as slow cooking root vegetables and pot herbs to warm your body instead of eating only salad.

In contrast, you can eat meats, eggs and drink milk once in a while. If you eat any food and drink too much, then you will be utilizing the glycolysis pathway dominantly, so the fundamental way to eat is to chew more and eat modestly. Eat until you're 80% full.

The foundation of my daily diets consists of brown rice and vegetables. By the way, it is fine not to be so strict and sensitive about it as well.

Your lifestyle does not need to lean extremely toward the mitochondrial pathway dominant lifestyle unless you are seeking to become a hermit.

Once in a while, you should enjoy eating or having drinks to relieve stress. That is also necessary for maintaining the balance between the body and soul.

Integrate Aerobic Exercise in Your Lifestyle

In addition to good eating habits, please integrate modest exercising to flee from the state of hypothermia and hypoxia. Exercising allows better blood circulation in our bodies.

However, we live in the modern age where many people do not need to move our bodies as they did in the past. It is a good idea to pick up some exercise routines and try them during the time you have between work and doing house chores. I do the following routines often:

■ **Arm Swing Exercise**
(While standing, swing both arms back and forth)

■ **8 Exercise**
(Hands in the air and try to write the number 8 with these hands in the air)

■ **Knee Bending and Stretching Exercise**
(Bend and stretch your knees rhythmically)

■ Body Swing
(While bending and stretching your knees, swing your body right and left)

In addition to these exercises, I go swimming since my house is by the beach. I also try to stay active by doing some routine house chores.

When you do light exercises, it allows oxygen flow through the body. As a result, the mitochondria become active and you feel energized. Try to incorporate some exercises at your own capacity. If you feel that you must exercise, then it becomes stressful and that is not good for your health.

In order to maintain a balance in your body, it is also important to build instantaneous force in addition to endurance. I build instantaneous force by practicing Karate kicks and hit baseballs at batting facilities. By doing these exercises, I try to use the energy produced by the glycolysis pathway as well.

4 Exercises Activate Mitochondria

■ Arm Swing Exercise

While standing, swing both arms back and forth

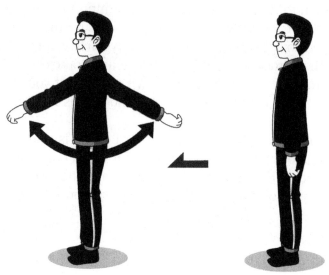

■ 8 Exercise

Hands in the air and try to write number 8 with these hands in the air

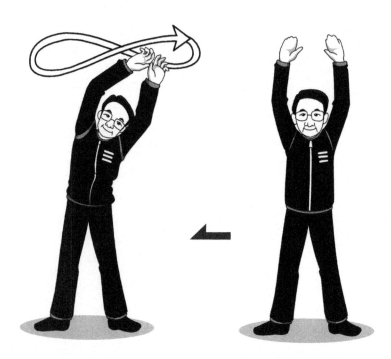

■ Knee Bending and Stretching Exercise

Bend and stretch your knees rhythmically, occasionally opening hip joints to repeat the same movements

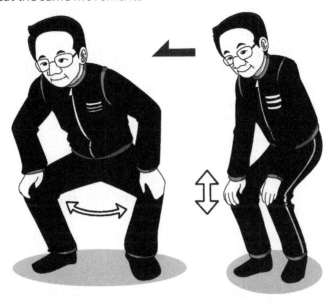

■ Body Swing

While bend and stretch your knees, swing your body right and left

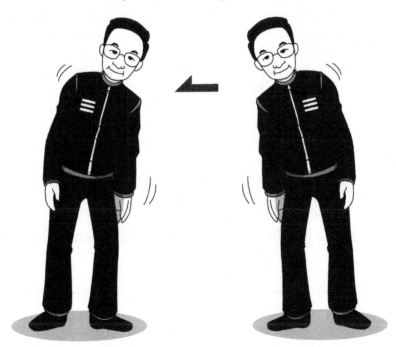

Cherish Good Laughs and Show Your Gratitude

As you grasp the tricks of handling stress and incorporating balanced daily diets and exercising, then the next step is to cherish good laughs and show your gratitude to others. It is widely known that laughing enhances the immune system as it makes the PNS dominant.

One experiment confirmed that laughing activated the NK (Natural Killer) cells which are one kind of the immune cells known to eliminate cancer cells. Laughing can lead you to a cancer free life.

Also, having a sense of gratitude can stimulate the PNS. This can also help to balance ourselves if your lifestyles are leaning toward the glycolysis pathway energy productions. If you are the kind of person who tends not to feel gratitude toward others, then start consciously using the words "Thank you" and "I appreciate it" more often.

When you get sick, try not to be pessimistic about it. Be positive and consider the sickness as an opportunity to re-examine your own lifestyle.

As I mentioned earlier, many cancer patients have a demeanor with furrowed brows.

To survive in this world, it is necessary to overcome challenges and get angry about injustices. However, it is also important to move on after feeling these emotions. If we all carry these feelings and anger all the time, then our bodies naturally will enter the conditions which induce cancer.

After expressing your feelings and having discussions, then move on and try not to carry those feelings with you.

You may feel some difficulties in practicing rules 1-6, but until you grasp the ability to incorporate these rules into your daily lives, please try them out step by step and at your own pace. You will notice that the mitochondrial pathway is being activated and as you continue, you will also be able to start to carry laughter and feelings of gratitude with you all the time.

Have a Purpose in Life, Find Joy in Your Lifetime and Set Goals

I still continue with my research even now and I
truly enjoy achieving big discoveries and having Aha! moments. Encountering these enjoyments and happiness in our own lives multiplies our strength to live, and create fuel to move on further.

Discovering the important concepts I have explained so far in my book, such as "all sicknesses are adaptive responses of our bodies" or "Cancer cells are not a failed function in our bodies", are results of building my life-long research one step at a time, and of continuing to pursue what I really love to do.

What we truly enjoy or our lifelong goals are not something you can think with your brain and find at once. By experiencing many things in our lives, while utilizing both energy powerhouses, the glycolysis pathway and the mitochondrial pathway in a balanced way, we can slowly discover these goals and what we truly enjoy in our lives.

At times in our lives, all of us encounter despair and suffer from severe stress. But, as long as you have a lifelong goal and something that you enjoy in your life as your foundation and in your core, you will be able to overcome these struggles positively. It is important to have a strong core and foundation – to live healthily.

Cancer free life parallels to life that is full of enjoyments and happiness. Let's get closer to this lifestyle. By understanding the true meaning of why we get illnesses, we can move forward to achieve the life full of happiness.

Epilogue - Realization by Understanding the Changes in the Body After Using a Hot Water Bottle

I clearly remember the day when I had a realization that led to a completely new theory about life, the theory I have explained in this book. It was late at night on January 10, 2008.

It was such a cold night, so I had many layers of blankets and a hot water bottle when I was sleeping.

I am a deep sleeper, so I usually sleep undisturbed until morning. But this evening, I woke up in the middle of the night.

When I look back, I then started to vaguely question the theory in my research. I felt like I was lacking something even though I was confident that the foundation of my research was correct and solid.

Perhaps, that affected my sleep. I looked at my skin where I was touching the hot water bottle while feeling sleepy headed. I saw that part of the skin became so thin. Also, I realized that my lower half did not feel energized.

Probably, people usually don't pay attention to such changes.

But, I was so intrigued by this bodily response that I could not fall asleep again. I kept thinking about this, and eventually it led me to the big realization.

It was the body's response where the mitochondrial pathway became dominant by warming the body, whereas in contrast, the glycolysis pathway slowed down which influenced the cell divisions.

Warming the body to activate the mitochondria is a secret to maintaining health. However, for men, energy produced in the glycolysis pathway is also important as sperm increase by cell divisions.

Cell divisions via the glycolysis pathways trigger the proliferation. When the glycolysis pathway becomes more dominant than the mitochondrial pathway, it encourages canceration. When we closely examine the Warburg effect, it leads us to such a conclusion.

When we look at this response of our bodies only, then we may conclude that the glycolysis pathway is a bad thing. But is that accurate? If we conclude that the glycolysis pathway is a bad pathway, then having cancer also means it is a bad thing for our bodies. I believe that everything that happens in our bodies has a reason, so we should understand the truth and wisdom of life in such a response of our bodies.

When I looked at the response from the understanding of life I have discovered and researched so far, then the glycolysis pathway which encourages the canceration has its place and role in life. It should have some meaning. This was when I gained the realization that having cancer is also an adaptive response. It was a moving moment, and the deep realization touched my heart greatly.

Under the conditions of hypothermia and hypoxia, the glycolysis pathway becomes dominant. Under these conditions, people get sick too. So, it is important to warm our bodies and take deep a breath to help the aerobic mitochondria become active.

But, it is also important to look at the other side of the coin. We need to see the reasons why people get sick. If we do not have an understanding of the reasons, then we may still be fixated on the idea that having sickness is a bad thing and may keep thinking that we need to remove the symptoms, which is the process typical to modern medicine.

The causes of diseases are only two things as I explained in my book: hypothermia and hypoxia. As you try to change your lifestyle while being attentive about eliminating the conditions of hypothermia and hypoxia, then spontaneous remission of cancer may be possible and various lifestyle-related diseases will diminish as well.

Please remember that diseases are caused while our bodies are trying to adapt to adverse internal conditions. It happens because our bodies found it necessary.

When we all gain this deep realization, it allows us to obtain balance in our life. It reminds us of how wonderful we are to live, and lets us feel that the positive and negative, ying and yang, can co-exist.

When you gain this realization of truth, you can reflect that upon your own lifestyle. You don't need to depend on others anymore, asking others to teach you and asking how to distinguish what is wrong. You can become independent by it and it will be a wisdom with which you can take control of your life.

If you are the kind of person who highly rate and trust modern medicine completely, then please refer to my book and try to re-examine how you live your life. There are only two causes of diseases. We can all practice the ways to escape from these two causes. It is a simple concept.

If you are the kind of person who is strict about certain diets and exercising, then please do not forget to seek balance in your life. I do not deny your practices, but I would like you to know that balance is important in life.

I believe that society will change when people realize the importance of having a balanced lifestyle. When that time comes, cancer will be considered as a common disease. The role of medicine in our daily lives will also be dramatically changed.

I wish that this book will trigger a change of thought in all of you, and become a starting point of making your life easier. Easier and happier in living our everyday lives.

July 2010,

Toru ABO

References

Journals/Thesis

Warburg, O. "On the origin of cancer cells" Science 123: 309-314, 1956.
Weinhouse, S. On respiratory impairment in cancer cells. Science 124: 267-269, 1956.
Sagan, L. On the origin of mitosing cells. Journal of Theoretical Biology 14: 255-274, 1967.
Sagiyama, K., Tsuchida, M., Kawamura, H., Wang, S., Li, C., Bai, X., Nagura, T., Nozoe, S. and Abo, T. Age-related bias in function of natural killer T cells and granulocytes after stress: reciprocal association of steroid hormones and sympathetic nerves. Clin. Exp. Immunol. 135: 56-63, 2004.
Tsuchida, M., Nagura, T., Bai. X., Li, C., Tomiyama-Miyaji, C., Kawamura, T., Uchiyama, M. and Abo T. Granulocytic activation and reciprocal immunosuppression induced by dehydration: relationship with renal failure. Biomed. Res. 25: 171-178, 2004.
Li, C., Bai, X., Wang, S., Tomiyama-Miyaji, C., Nagura, T., Kawamura, T.and Abo, T. Immunopotentiation of NKT cells by low-protein diet and the suppressive effect on tumor metastasis. Cell. Immunol. 231: 96-102, 2004.
Abo, T., Kawamura, T. and Watanabe, H. Immunologic states of autoimmune diseases. Immnologic Res. 33: 23-34, 2005.
Ariyasinghe, A., Morshed, S.R.M., Mannoor, M.K., Bakir, H.Y., Kawamura, H., Miyaji, C., Nagura, T., Kawamura, T., Watanabe, H., Sekikawa, H. and Abo, T. Protection against malaria due to innate immunity enhanced by low-protein diet. J. Parasitol. 92: 531-538, 2006.
Ren, HW., Shen, JW., Tomiyama-Miyaji, C., Watanabe, M., Kainuma, E., Inoue, M., Kuwano, Y. and Abo, T. Augmentation of innate immunity by low-dose irradiation. Cell. Immunol. 244:50-56, 2006.
Abo, T., Kawamura, T., Kawamura, H., Tomiyama-Miyaji, C. and Kanda, Y. Relationship between diseases accompanied by tissue destruction and granulocytes with surface adrenergic receptors. Immunologic Res. 37: 201-210, 2007.
Tomiyama-Miyaji, C., Watanabe, M., Ohishi, T., Kanda, Y., Kainuma, E., Bakir, H.Y., Shen, JW., Ren, HW., Inoue, M., Tajima, K., Bai, X. and Abo, T. Modulation of the endocrine and immune systems by well-controlled hyperthermia equipment. Biomed. Res. 28: 119-125, 2007.
Watanabe, M., Tomiyama-Miyaji, C., Kainuma, E., Inoue, M., Kuwano, Y., Ren, HW., Shen, JW. and Abo, T. Role of α adrenergic stimulus in stress-

induced modulation of body temperature, blood glucose and innate immunity. Immunol. Lett. 115: 43-49, 2008.

Tachikawa, S., Kawamura, T., Kawamura, H., Kanda, Y., Fujii, Y., Matsumoto, H. and Abo, T. Appearance of B220 [low] autoantibody-producing B-1 cells at neonatal and older stages in mice. Clin. Exp. Immunol. 153: 448-455, 2008.

Kainuma, E., Watanabe, M., Tomiyama-Miyaji, C., Inoue, M., Kuwano, Y., Ren, HW. and Abo, T. Proposal of alternative mechanism responsible for the function of high-speed swimsuits. Biomed. Res. 30: 69-70, 2009.

Ohishi, T., Nukuzuma, C., Seki, A., Watanabe, M., Tomiyama-Miyaji, C., Kainuma, E., Inoue, M., Kuwano, Y. and Abo, T. Alkalization of blood pH is responsible for survival of cancer patients by mild hyperthermia. Biomed. Res. 30: 95-100, 2009.

Kainuma, E., Watanabe, M., Tomiyama-Miyaji, C., Inoue, M., Kuwano, Y., Ren, HW. and Abo, T. Association of glucocorticoid with stress-induced modulation of body temperature, blood glucose and innate immunity. Psychoneuroendocrinol. 34:1459-1468, 2009

Shen, JW., Ren, HW., Tomiyama-Miyaji, C., Watanabe, M., Kainuma, E., Inoue, M., Kuwano, Y. and Abo, T. Resistance and augmentation of innate immunity in mice exposed to starvation. Cell. Immunol. 259: 66-73, 2009.

Books

Luckey, T.D. 『Hormesis with Ionizing Radiation』 CRC, Boca Raton Press, Florida, 1980, ISBN-13: 978-0849358418

Luckey, T.D. Radiation Hormesis, CRC Press, Boca Raton Press, Florida, 1991,
ISBN-13: 978-0849361593, In Japanese, Soft Science Inc., Tokyo, 1993 ISBN-13: 978-4881710487.

Lane, N., Power, Sex, Suicide: Mitochondria and the
Meaning of Life, Oxford University Press, UK, ISBN-13: 978-0192804815, 2005,
In Japanese, Misuzu Shobo, Tokyo, 2007, ISBN-13: 978-0199205646

Sena, H., Ota, N., 『Mitokondoria no Chikara』 Shincho Bunko Tokyo, 2007, ISBN-13: 978-4101214351

Voet, D. and Voet, J.G., Glycolysis. In: D. Voet, J.G. Voet,
Eds., Biochemistry, 3rd Edition, J. Wiley & Sons, New York, 2004, ISBN-13: 978-0471193500

Kono, S., 「Mitokondoria no Nazo」Kodansha, Tokyo, 1999, ISBN-13: 978-4061494558

Kuroiwa, T., 「Mitokondoria ha Dokokara Kitaka Seimei
40 Oku Nen wo Sakanoboru」Nihon Hoso Shuppan Kyokai, Tokyo, 2000, ISBN-13: 978-4140018873

Hayashi, J., 「Mitokondoria Misteri Odorokubeki Saibou
Syoukikan no Hataraki」Kodansha, Tokyo, 2002, ISBN-13: 978-4062573917

Sena, H., Ota, N., 「Mitokondoria to Ikiru」 Kadokawa
Shoten, Tokyo, 2000, ISBN-13: 978-4047040069

Utsumi, K., Inoue, M. translation supervisor, 「Shin Mitokondoria Gaku」
Kyoritsu Syuppan, Tokyo, 2001, ISBN-13: 978-4320055810

Kuroki, T., 「Kenkou・Rouka・Jumyo Hito to Inochi no Bunkashi」Chuou Kouronsha, Tokyo, 2007, ISBN-13: 978-4121018984

Oyama, T. translation supervisor, 「Be-shikku Masuta Seikagaku」Ohm-sha, Tokyo, 2008, ISBN-13: 978-4274206047

Knoll, A.H., Life on a Young Planet: The First Three Billion Years of Evolution on Earth, Princeton University Press, N.J., 2004 , ISBN-13: 978-4314009881, In Japanese, Kinokuniya Shoten, Tokyo, 2005, , ISBN-13: 978-4314009881.

Ishikawa, H., et al., 「Siri-zu Shinkagaku 3 Kagakushinka・Saibou Shinka」 Iwanami Shoten, 2004, Tokyo, ISBN-13: 978-4000069236

Weinberg, R., The Biology of Cancer, Garland Science, UK, 2006, ISBN-13: 978-0815340768

Weinberg, R., One Renegade Cell: How Cancer Begins, Basic Books, N.Y., 1999, ISBN-13: 978-0465072767 In Japanese, Soushisha, Tokyo, 1999, ISBN-13: 978-4794209238

Abo, T., 「Iryou ga Yamai wo Tsukuru Meneki karano Keisyo」Iwanami Shoten, Tokyo, 2001, ISBN-13: 978-4000221139

Abo , T., 「Meneki Shinkaron」Kawade yobo Shinsha , Tokyo, 2006, ISBN-13: 978-4309409559

Abo , T., 「Byoki ha Jibun de Naosu Menekigaku 101 no Syohousen」Shinchosha, Tokyo, 2006, ISBN-13: 978-4101350318

Iriki, M., 「Taion Seirigaku Tekisuto - Wakariyasui Taion no Ohanashi -」Bunkoudo, Tokyo, 2003, ISBN-13: 978-4830602207

NHK reporting team., 「Seimei 40 Okunen Harukana Tabi 1 - 5」Nihon Hoso Syuppan Kyokai, Tokyo, 1994 - 95, ISBN-13: 978-4140809044

Inoue M., translation supervisor 「Saito Purotekusyon (Cytoprotection) – Seitai Bougyo Kikou no Genryu wo Saguru」 Gan to Kagaku Ryohosha,

Tokyo, 2002, ISBN-13: 978-4906225378

Ward, P.D., Out of Thin Air: Dinosaurs, Birds, and Earth's Ancient Atmosphere, Joseph Henry Press; 1ˢᵗ Edition, 2006, Washington DC, ISBN-13: 978-0309100618 In Japanese, Bungei Syunju Press, Tokyo 2008, ISBN-13: 978-4163699608

Toru Abo, M.D., Ph.D. Dr. Abo was born in 1947 in Minmaya village of Aomori Prefecture, Japan. He received his medical degree from the Tohoku University of Medicine in 1972. He currently serves as a Professor at Niigata University, Graduate School of Medical and Dental Science Research, and at the Department of Immunology and Medical Zoology. His significant discoveries include the creation of a monoclonal antibody against NK cell antigen CD57 while attending Alabama University in 1980, which he named "Len-7". He discovered "extrathymic T cells" in 1989 and uncovered the solution to "the mechanism of white blood cells controlled by the autonomic nervous system" in 1996, all vital discoveries that surprised the world. He is also the author of a number of books, including "Your Immune Revolution (Kodansha International)" and "Self-Cure Sickness (Shinchosha)". He co-authored numerous publications as well, including "Lifestyle Chases Cancer Away" and "Lifestyle Chases Diseases Away", both by Makino Shuppann.

CPSIA information can be obtained
at www.ICGtesting.com
Printed in the USA
BVOW06s1929191017
498174BV00013B/73/P